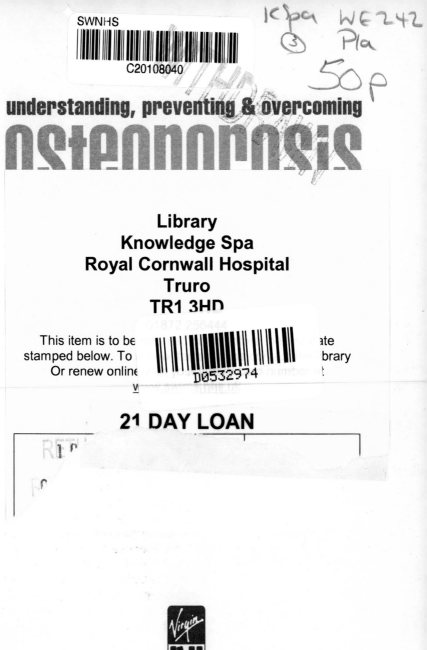

Kpa WE242
③ Pla

50p

understanding, preventing & overcoming
OSTEOPOROSIS

This edition published in Great Britain in 2004 by
Virgin Books Ltd
Thames Wharf Studios
Rainville Road
London
W6 9HA

First published in hardback in 2003 by Virgin Books Ltd

A catalogue record for this book is available
from the British Library.

ISBN 0 7535 0893 1

Typeset by Phoenix Photosetting, Chatham, Kent
Printed and bound in Great Britain by
Mackays of Chatham, Chatham, Kent

Contents

Acknowledgements

Jane and Gill would like to thank their husbands, Peter Simpson and David Falvey, for their encouragement, support and practical help with the book. They also wish to thank Henry Haslam for his assistance with research for the book.

Introduction

Until man can produce a blade of grass, nature can laugh at his so-called scientific knowledge. Remedies from chemicals will never stand in favour compared with the products of nature, the living cell of the plant and the final result of the rays of the sun, the mother of all life.

Thomas A. Edison

WELCOME

You may have picked up this book because:
● You suffer from osteoporosis
● You know someone or look after someone who suffers from osteoporosis and you want to help them
● One of your parents or close relatives suffers from the disease and you fear that in the future it will affect you

By opening this book, you have taken the first step in taking control of osteoporosis and its effects on your life and those dear to you. By reading the book and following the dietary and lifestyle advice it contains, we believe that most of you will be able to prevent yourselves from ever suffering from the disease. We also believe that those of you already suffering from osteoporosis will greatly improve your chances of increasing your bone strength and health, treating the disease, and regaining control of your lives.

We reject the conventional Western medical view that the disease is an inevitable part of ageing. We also challenge much of the orthodox prevention and treatment regimes promulgated in books, leaflets and websites by individual authors and by national institutes and charities concerned with osteoporosis. These typically recommend a diet high in calcium, especially from dairy produce, vitamin D and other supplementation and medication which, in the case of post-menopausal women, is frequently hormone replacement therapy. All of this is aimed at merely slowing bone loss, rather than restoring bone health.

Looking at the health outcomes of our many friends and colleagues with osteoporosis who have followed such advice, and at official predictions of future increases in the disease, it appears that such an approach on its own is powerless to protect us from the so-called 'silent epidemic' of osteoporosis.

In this book we take a radically different approach, based on studies and analysis of mainstream scientific literature. Our scientific training has taught us to observe and record objectively, to root out every fragment of information, to sift the relevant from the irrelevant, the rational from the irrational – and to do so with a healthy scepticism of science funded by organisations with a vested interest in obtaining a particular result.

We tell you how to get the best out of orthodox medicine. We also tell you about medications which, when used to treat other illnesses, ranging from allergies to cancer, can actually cause osteoporosis. We give you a new dietary regime of delicious nutritious recipes, based on the traditional dietary principles of China, where the rate of osteoporosis is forty to fifty times lower than that of rich, industrialised countries such as Germany, the UK and the USA. We include advice on obtaining the micronutrients that are essential for bone health, how to avoid bone-damaging pollutants, and which forms of exercise are suitable for different stages of osteoporosis, ages and personalities – and much more.

How can we speak with such confidence? Because we have had experience of using dietary and lifestyle factors, based on sound science, to prevent, control and treat equally distressing and dangerous illnesses, most notably breast cancer.

Jane's own experience of breast cancer, which recurred four times after her initial mastectomy and involved her in four further operations, 35 radiotherapy treatments, irradiation of her ovaries to induce menopause and twelve chemotherapy treatments, is published in her international bestseller *Your Life in Your Hands*.[1] This book tells how she used her scientific knowledge and experience of working in China to identify dairy produce as the principal factor promoting her breast cancer. Within five weeks of eliminating all dairy produce from her otherwise healthy diet and lifestyle, a large secondary tumour in her neck had totally disappeared, and she has been free of cancer for ten years.

Your Life in Your Hands explores the epidemiological evidence connecting breast (and prostate) cancer with dairy consumption, as well as emerging, but nonetheless hard, scientific evidence in support of such a connection. It goes on to develop a diet and lifestyle based on seven food factors and five lifestyle factors (including eliminating all dairy produce) – a regime called 'The Plant Programme'. With her friend and fellow scientist, Gill Tidey, this was expanded in a second book, *The Plant Programme*,[2] which provides new evidence of the importance of diet in the prevention of cancer and other diseases and contains a large number of recipes for delicious, nutritious meals. *Your Life in Your Hands* is about why you should change your diet and lifestyle: *The Plant Programme* is about how to achieve this.*

The Plant Programme also has a message for the sceptics. We said, in effect, 'Well, even if you are not totally convinced of the arguments in the books, when you can eat so well by following the regime, especially eliminating dairy, why not?' In science, such an approach is known as the 'precautionary principle', and it is often put into effect in our everyday lives to reduce various risks.

Together, we have received hundreds of letters, phone calls and e-mails about our two books, mostly from people who have followed our advice and whose cancer (breast, prostate and some other types of the disease) is now in remission. Many readers have also told us how the advice has cured allergic conditions such as asthma and eczema, other skin problems such as psoriasis, and digestive problems including Crohn's disease and irritable bowel syndrome. Closer to home, Jane's husband Peter has experienced great improvement in his osteoarthritis since adopting the regime and no longer needs

---

* The diet and lifestyle described in this book and in *Your Life in Your Hands* and *The Plant Programme* are meant to complement, not replace, orthodox medicine. Before making any changes, discuss the new evidence presented with your doctor.

any pain-killing or other medication. All agree that their health has improved by following the Plant Programme.

Increasingly, we hear of medical professionals recommending the books *Your Life in Your Hands* and *The Plant Programme* to their patients, and they are now included in self-help packs provided by some general medical practices for their breast and prostate cancer patients. Increasingly, too, supermarkets and small shops are marketing and promoting dairy-free and other produce recommended in the Plant Programme.

THE TRIUMPH OF ADVERTISING OVER SCIENCE

In spite of the Plant Programme's success in helping to treat (and, hopefully, prevent) breast and prostate cancer and other conditions, many people have expressed concern about the possible effect of the diet on their bones and their risk of developing osteoporosis. The most commonly asked questions are 'Won't I get osteoporosis?' or 'Won't my osteoporosis get worse if I stop eating dairy products?' or 'Where do I get my calcium from?' The marketing of dairy produce as an essential source of calcium has been so strong that even some medical professionals, who should know better, insist that eliminating dairy produce from the diet will lead to calcium deficiency and hence increase the risk of osteoporosis. In this book, we present evidence, from the peer-reviewed scientific literature, which strongly and convincingly refutes this. Indeed, we believe that we show that this is one of the great myths of our time!

While we have always been fully confident that our diet provides good sources of bio-available calcium, we have researched the subject further and found compelling evidence in the scientific literature that it is the Western diet and lifestyle that are at the root of the problem. Far from being beneficial, the consumption of dairy products, especially cheese, is actually damaging to those at risk from osteoporosis and other bone disease. **For many people, cheese is likely to be part of the cause, not the cure, of osteoporosis.**

However, the answer to osteoporosis is not as simple as just giving up dairy products. This book takes you through the detail of a whole new diet and lifestyle, with seven Food Factors and eight Lifestyle Factors (the 'Osteoporosis Plant Programme'), which will improve your bone health, appearance and outlook. The Osteoporosis Plant Programme is based on the Plant Programme, adapted particularly to improve bone health.

The extent and impact of osteoporosis are alarming. One in three women and one in twelve men over the age of fifty in the UK already suffer from the condition, and every three minutes someone has a fracture due to osteoporosis.[3] In the USA it is predicted that one in two women and one in eight men over fifty will have an osteoporosis-related fracture at some time in their lives. In Canada, more women die each year as a result of osteoporotic fractures than from breast and ovarian cancer combined.[4] Just as in the case of breast and prostate cancer, the statistics on the rate of osteoporosis are stark and shocking – and initially frightening. However, we believe that, as with breast and prostate cancer, we can set before you, clearly and plainly, vital information from the mainstream scientific literature which can help you to cut drastically your risk of suffering from osteoporosis or from suffering further bone degeneration if you are already affected by the disease.

As in our earlier books on breast and prostate cancer, our aim is to present a diet and lifestyle that will empower you to fight osteoporosis, and help you to work with your doctor to help yourself.

One of the great fears that surrounds osteoporosis is that the condition is irreversible and, once someone has it, bones cannot be regenerated. Unfortunately, this is probably true for some individuals, although further degeneration can be prevented. On the other hand, scientific evidence from the US National Aeronautics and Space Administration (NASA) on the demineralisation and remineralisation of the bones of astronauts during and after space missions suggests that many people may be helped greatly by changing their diet and lifestyle. Evidence to support this view also comes from studies of people suffering from a condition called hyperparathyroidism. This condition causes serious calcium loss from the bones until the condition is treated, following which the bones are remineralised.

The Osteoporosis Plant Programme diet is rich in plant proteins, essential fatty acids, fibre, phyto-oestrogens, vitamins and minerals, including calcium, and much published research discussed in this book indicates that such a diet is protective against osteoporosis. The new information is strongly supported by epidemiological evidence which clearly shows that, like breast and prostate cancer, osteoporosis is mainly a disease of rich Western countries where people consume a diet that includes large quantities of animal protein (especially dairy produce and meat) and junk food and drink, with too little or inappropriate exercise.

We can almost hear those of you who have not read *Your Life in Your Hands* and *The Plant Programme* asking, 'Is this just another diet to add to all the other supposedly healthy diets being promoted in books, videos and the media?' There are so many out there: the so-called detoxifying diets, the fat-burning and the food-combining diets – often started and promoted by individual scientists or medical professionals, including dieticians, and then copied and quoted until the next one comes along. One of the difficulties for most people is that the advice given in different books is often conflicting: whereas one diet recommends eating lots of complex carbohydrates, another diet suggests that some such foods trigger a rise in blood-sugar levels and should be avoided or, at least, limited.

Some diets recommend eating lots of animal protein while others recommend cutting it out completely. It is usually difficult, if not impossible, to check the scientific basis of the recommended diets, because the scientific papers on which they are based are not included or are not attached to particular statements. One best-selling supposedly anti-cancer diet we read recently recommended meat and dairy produce (advice we strongly refute in *Your Life in Your Hands* and *The Plant Programme*). Anything good in dairy produce, whether calcium or the now highly promoted conjugated linoleic acids (CLAs), comes from plants or the action on them of microbes in the gut. Surely it is better to eat salads and vegetables that are not unlike the grasses that are eaten by cows in the first place – after all, they are the real source of the immensely strong bones of cows and hippopotamuses!

Other diet books begin by strongly recommending the elimination of all dairy produce or wheat, for example, but then actually include lots of recipes containing these ingredients.

Our work is different. We are both natural scientists – trained to consider the complexity of the real world and to search for fundamental processes to explain natural phenomena such as earthquakes and volcanoes. Similarly, our approach to understanding the origins of disease is based on fundamental causative factors. This is a radically different approach to that of many medical researchers, whose work is mainly directed towards finding pills and potions to treat symptoms. Let us illustrate this fundamental difference of approach:

Jane has worked on environmental geochemistry for much of her career. This has involved her and her team in studying concentrations of chemical elements in the environment that are so high that they are toxic, or so low that they cause deficiency conditions. Such geochemical anomalies in soils and water can be related to specific diseases in people who eat foods grown in such soils or drink the affected water. To take a couple of examples, by the mid-1960s the levels of the trace element cadmium were so high in the Jinzu River Basin in Toyama, Japan, that people consuming local food and water suffered severe skeletal problems with the development of a painful disease known as 'Itai-Itai' (translated 'Ouch-Ouch') disease. Elsewhere in continental Asia, low concentrations of the trace elements selenium and iodine are associated with serious skeletal problems resulting in bone deformation ('Big Bone disease'). What has been demonstrated, time and again, by this type of environmental study is that until the fundamental cause of such problems is identified there is little or nothing that can be done to help the affected individuals by way of pills and potions or to stop the disease recurring. Until you have found the underlying cause or causes (whether it is bone or any other disease) and effectively neutralised it, you cannot claim to have dealt with the problem.

Gill's scientific career has been marked by a different kind of search for fundamental explanations. As a micropalaeontologist working for the oil exploration industry in south-east Asia, her job was to identify and determine the age of very small fossils that occur in sedimentary rocks. This painstaking task was carried out while an exploration well was actually being drilled, and accurate dating of the layers of rocks through which drilling was taking place was crucial. Gill discovered early in her career that it was absolutely essential to consider the whole assemblage of fossil evidence, and never to jump to quick conclusions based on partial evidence, no matter how compelling.

As scientists we feel that it is essential to develop our diet and lifestyle recommendations based on similar sound science using information from the mainstream peer-reviewed literature and to give the sources of the information we use. Also, instead of simply buying recipes we have worked closely together to develop dishes which follow the scientific principles spelled out in the book, and which are also delicious to eat. There is nothing extreme or dangerous in our diet: it is not based on single-issue science such as the amount of insulin release triggered by different foods. Instead, it is based on the principles of the Chinese diet. A healthy diet involves many complex factors, and the traditional Chinese diet has been evolved over many centuries by one of the most biologically successful peoples on Earth, using sustainable agricultural practices. It is an agricultural and dietary philosophy that has been studied in detail by a team of eminent scientists from Cornell, Oxford and Beijing universities during the 1980s, who showed its great health benefits.[5]

The contrast between the progressive evolution of the traditional Chinese approach and the Western approach of discarding the old in favour of the latest fad is illustrated by the following:

A Short History of Medicine[6]

Doctor, I have an earache:

2000 BC	Here, eat this root.
AD 1000	That root is heathen. Here, say this prayer.
AD 1850	That prayer is supersition. Here, drink this potion.
AD 1940	That potion is snakeoil. Here, swallow this pill.
AD 1985	That pill is ineffective. Here, take this antibiotic.
AD 2000	That antibiotic is artificial. Here, eat this root.

HOW TO USE THIS BOOK

Before you begin, it might help if we give you a few tips on how to use the book. The book comprises two main sections. The first seven chapters, forming Section 1, are about understanding, preventing and treating osteoporosis from a scientific perspective. Section 2 is a cookbook packed with delicious bone-healthy recipes.

If you simply want to prevent or treat osteoporosis you may wish to begin by reading Chapters 5 and 6 and following the straightforward advice on diet and lifestyle given there and in Section 2. The recommended diet is based on principles borrowed from Asia, especially China.

If, on the other hand, you wish to explore in greater depth and understand the basis for this advice, you should begin at Chapter 2 and follow the argument through. We hope to take you through the scientific detective story and to answer the two key questions that are at the heart of scientific endeavour – 'Why?' and 'How?': *why* does this disease affect increasing numbers of people, and *how* can people equip themselves to prevent and treat it?

In Chapter 1 we take you through the diagnosis and treatment of osteoporosis by orthodox medicine, as seen through the experiences of friends and colleagues who suffer from the disease. Treatment has typically involved consuming large quantities of dairy produce in the diet, taking calcium and other supplements such as magnesium and vitamin D, frequently combined with hormone replacement therapy for post-menopausal women. Much of this conventional wisdom is challenged later in the book.

Chapters 2 to 4 form the 'why' section of the book. In Chapter 2, we review what osteoporosis is, with particular reference to the role of the skeleton and bones in the human body. The skeleton is not only an amazing structural support system for the body; it is also the body's principal store of calcium and other alkaline minerals and bases such as bicarbonates, which can be released into the bloodstream as the body's first line of defence in neutralising or buffering excess acid build-up. In Chapter 3 we consider what the mainstream scientific literature has to say about the real causes of the disease. The chapter includes epidemiological evidence on the distribution of osteoporotic disease in relation to diet in 33 countries of the world. This evidence is considered in the light of the latest scientific information on the processes in the body that can cause bone degeneration and hence osteoporosis, particularly excess acidity generated by poor diets, stress and other lifestyle factors typical of Western industrialised countries.

Chapter 4 provides a simple, clear explanation of the latest scientific evidence on which foods and activities produce acidity or alkalinity in the body. Emphasis is placed on achieving a proper balance because, although bone damage is strongly linked to excess acidity, excess alkalinity in the body can cause other types of ill health. The importance of levels of 'good' trace elements, such as zinc and copper, in maintaining bone health is also considered. The chapter includes a table listing many common foodstuffs against their acidity rating when metabolised in the body; another table lists the calcium and magnesium contents of these foods. These tables will help you to plan your diet to protect against bone degeneration. The chapter also provides information on how to obtain essential nutrients from food, without the need to resort to man-made mineral and vitamin supplements.

The next part of the book (Chapters 5 and 6) is the 'how' section. It develops simple dietary and lifestyle factors based on the scientific evidence in the early chapters of the book. In Chapter 6, we provide sound lifestyle tips – for example how natural herbal methods can be substituted for hormone replacement therapy, what is a sensible amount of alcohol to consume, why and how to reduce cigarette smoking, how to limit your exposure to substances such as cadmium and other pollutants which are harmful to bones, types of medication to be concerned about and appropriate exercise.

In Chapter 7, we consider why we continue to be fed all the wrong messages by the popular media and many medical professionals. Is there really a conspiracy between the dairy industry, calcium and vitamin supplement manufacturers, those marketing hormone replacement therapy and Dual X-ray Absorptiometry (DEXA) machines, some charities and the medical profession? We discover what we, as individuals, can do to help ourselves and reduce our exposure, as a society, to the appalling human, social and economic costs of the so-called 'silent epidemic' of osteoporosis.

In the second major section of the book we provide you with the 'Osteoporosis Plant Programme' Cookbook. This includes more than 100 recipes for delicious meals that are protective of bone and good for health generally. As in *The Plant Programme*, these meals are based on using healthy, nutritious ingredients to prepare dishes that are tempting and delicious. The recipes are simple, practical and easy to follow, and are mostly inexpensive and quick to make.

Finally we should like to assure you that we have no agenda driven by factors such as funding from vested-interest groups to promote particular foods or other products and that we have, as far as possible, tried to identify and eliminate such biased sources of information from our work.

1 Bones of Contention

In this chapter we look at the orthodox medical approach to osteoporosis (originally known as 'brittle bone disease') through the eyes and experiences of some of our friends, colleagues and associates afflicted by it. We look at the way the World Health Organisation (WHO) has developed the use of measured bone mineral density to estimate the risk of fracture due to osteoporosis. We then review the much-repeated risk factors for low bone mineral density and osteoporosis, and the recommended preventative measures promulgated by leading medical professionals and charities.[1, 2, 3] By observing the treatment and health outcomes of our many friends and colleagues with osteoporosis and reading the official predictions of the future impact of the disease, we are led to conclude that conventional medicine on its own appears powerless to protect us against the 'silent epidemic' of osteoporosis.

Our two previous books, *Your Life in Your Hands*[4] and *The Plant Programme*,[5] were written from personal experience of successfully battling with potentially life-threatening disease against the odds – in Jane's case five episodes of breast cancer and in Gill's case a diagnosis of pre-cancerous calcification of the breasts. However, neither of us has any personal experience of osteoporosis (or brittle bone disease).

Jane, now in her late fifties, continues to do geological field visits as part of her job and her collisions with rocks are often to be seen recorded in the bruises on her arms and legs. Gill is in her mid-fifties and, while no longer a professional geologist, is an active, handicap-12 golfer, and often plays in regional and county matches. Both of us tend to dash around the UK and other countries wearing high-heeled shoes and carrying heavy luggage (mostly comprising weighty committee papers and reports, or sets of golf clubs and related paraphernalia). This is behaviour guaranteed to put great stress on the bones and skeleton, especially the hip joint and back. Yet neither of us has suffered any serious pain, or other problems associated with our bones or skeletons that the occasional visit to the osteopath has not dealt with.

Contrast this with the situation of one of our friends, Joanne (not her real name), a former headmistress turned civil servant, who a few years ago (then in her mid-fifties) was walking across her carpeted office wearing sensible flat-heeled shoes carrying only a thin file. Suddenly and quite unexpectedly she fell to the floor in severe pain. She was rushed to hospital and diagnosed with a fractured hip. She was in plaster and forced to walk on crutches for many weeks. After a series of tests she was told that she was suffering from osteoporosis and that this was why her hip had fractured. **Put more starkly, Joanne had not fallen and fractured her hip – her hip had fractured, and she had fallen down.**

We both have many women friends and acquaintances in their fifties and over. Because osteoporosis is now so common (see page IX), we know many women diagnosed with the disease. They are, by and large, sensible, independent women who have or have had professional careers. They know all the conventional wisdom on risk factors and preventative measures about osteoporosis and they try to help themselves and take charge of their health. Many of them feel the same sense of anger and frustration that Jane felt when she was first diagnosed with breast cancer. They all, in one way or another, want an answer to the question, 'Why me?' – especially when they believe they have been very responsible about their health.

Take the case of Mary (a combination of several people), an executive in a hospital trust. She is always beautifully groomed. She exercises regularly and often has a slight tan from skiing or other outdoor pursuits. She has never smoked and has only an occasional glass of wine with a meal out. She has hardly been ill in her life and was totally shocked when, aged 54, she attended an executive health check organised by her employers and was told that she had severe osteoporosis in both of her hips and lower spine.

Harriet (also a combination of several people), a nurse who is married to a doctor, was first diagnosed as suffering from osteoporosis when she began to complain of severe indigestion and breathlessness. Tests revealed that the problems were being caused by the changing shape of her spine which was compressing her lungs, stomach and other organs of her digestive tract as a result of osteoporosis. Despite following the best medical advice available, she has now, in her early seventies, lost height and has a clearly developed 'Dowager's Hump' (more grandly termed 'kyphosis' by conventional medicine). This is caused by the shortening and curvature of her upper spine (symptoms thought to be the result of multiple fractures of the spinal vertebrae)[6]. She even has problems with her teeth, which her dentist is working hard to keep aligned.

We know hardly any men with the disease, probably because fewer of them are affected by it. This is thought to be because the physiological and hormonal differences between males and females mean osteoporosis affects a much higher proportion of women than men. Although we have not been able to discuss their illness with our two former colleagues who have been diagnosed with osteoporosis (remember – Men are from Mars) we are aware that they had to give up their jobs and it was most noticeable that they lost height over a relatively short period of time – a few months in one case.

Before we try to answer the 'why me?' question for these and other sufferers of osteoporosis, let us look at the illness and its formal definition by the World Health Organisation (WHO). Let us also look at the conventional risk factors for osteoporosis according to orthodox medicine, and at the diagnosis, treatment and advice on prevention that is given to sufferers by national agencies, charities and other organisations concerned with osteoporosis.[7, 8, 9]

WHAT IS OSTEOPOROSIS?

Osteoporosis is a disease characterised by low bone mass and deterioration of bone tissue, leading to increased bone fragility and risk of fracture, particularly of the hip, spine and wrist. Osteoporosis has been called the 'silent disease' because bone loss occurs initially without symptoms. People may not know that they have osteoporosis until, as in Joanne's case, their bones become so weak that a sudden strain, bump, fall or movement causes a hip to fracture, or a vertebra to collapse. Collapsed vertebrae may initially be felt as severe back pain or other symptoms caused by compression of internal organs by a collapsing, curving spine, as was the case with Harriet, or they may become apparent in a loss of height, spinal deformities, or severely stooped posture.

The WHO has developed specific criteria for osteoporosis, whereby the risk of bone fracture depends on the measurement of bone mineral density. In 1991, a panel of experts defined osteoporosis as 'a systemic disease characterised by low bone mass and microarchitectural deterioration of the skeleton, leading to enhanced bone fragility and increased fracture risk'.[10] This definition is based on two of the skeletal changes considered to be most important in osteoporosis – the diminished bone mass and the diminished bone quality. At the time, however, the definition was considered impractical, since the only means of assessing bone quality then was the study of samples of bone (removed surgically), a procedure which was costly and did not lend itself to periodic monitoring.

In 1994, following the introduction of new methods of measuring bone density, a new WHO panel of experts defined 'low bone mass' more precisely.[11] The group began by agreeing two basic concepts. First, they assumed that fracture risk must be lowest when bone mineral density is highest – some time between ages twenty and forty in healthy people. The standard average bone mineral density was based on results obtained on a specially selected group or sample of 25-year-old Caucasian women (i.e. white women of European descent). The relative risk for fracture in this standard reference group was arbitrarily set at 1.0. Secondly, the expert panel agreed, on the basis of several studies,[12] that the relative risk for fracture increases as bone mineral density decreases, and that the relationship between bone mineral density and fracture risk is continuous and there is no fracture threshold. Thus, patients with a bone mineral density score significantly below the mean for peak bone mass are considered to be at increased risk of bone fracture.

For someone with a score of –2, the risk of suffering an osteoporosis-related fracture is considered double that of someone with the same bone mineral density as the average of the WHO sample. A score of –4 doubles the risk again, to four times that of those individuals with 'normal' bone density.

The fact that the WHO sample consisted entirely of Caucasians has led to criticism of the basis of the method and its general diagnostic value. The use of bone mineral density has also been criticised[13] on the basis that the density can vary depending on the size of a woman's bones as well as on the concentration of minerals in the bone. Because a larger person generally has larger bones than a smaller person does, the energy beam will encounter more minerals in a large person's bones than in a small person's of the same density. Hence, even if the true densities of both bones are identical, DEXA or DPA tests will indicate a higher 'density' in a large-boned than a small-boned person. Thus, it is argued, there are no bone mineral density levels that are 'high', 'low' or 'normal' for everyone. What is normal for one woman may be low or high for another. Nevertheless, despite any shortcomings of bone mineral density testing, it is valuable as an index of changes (either deterioration or improvement) in bone mineral density over time, provided that the same equipment is used on each occasion.

TESTING FOR OSTEOPOROSIS

The most common test, Dual Energy X-ray Absorptiometry (DEXA or DXA) is usually used to scan the bones of the lower back and hips. The machine produces a printout that compares your bone density with that of the average obtained on the WHO sample of young white women. The difference between your bone density and this average is then calculated to give a score. Scores between 0 (no difference from the average) and –1 are considered normal. Scores between –1 and –2.5 are diagnosed as suffering from osteopenia, or at increased risk of osteoporosis. Where scores are below –2.5, patients are diagnosed as having osteoporosis.

For those of you who are more mathematically inclined, the scores are standard deviations (or average differences from the average).

See below for more information on this and other diagnostic methods.

This new WHO definition of osteoporosis moved the disorder from a disease of fractures, to a disease of fracture *risk*. Just as high blood lipids (fatty substances) and blood pressure are indicators of a risk of heart disease, so bone mineral density is now viewed as a predictor of osteoporosis.

RECEIVED WISDOM

The orthodox medical view is that there is no single cause of osteoporosis, which can be due to decreased bone formation in early life, or to increased bone loss later in life. Before we follow the stories of Joanne, Mary and Harriet further, and consider why they might have been at particular risk of developing osteoporosis, let us look at the risk factors for the disease according to conventional medicine.

Some of these (based mainly on information from the US National Institute of Health, Osteoporosis,[14] the Osteoporosis Society of Canada[15] and the National Osteoporosis Society in the UK,[16] and from Goddard and Kleerekoper[17]) are given below. We note where we agree with or challenge the orthodox medical view.

RISK FACTORS THAT YOU CANNOT CHANGE

Gender	Your chances of developing osteoporosis are greater if you are a woman. Women have less bone tissue and lose bone more rapidly than men because of hormonal changes, especially the decline in oestrogen levels after the menopause.	**AGREED**
Age	The older you are, the greater your risk of osteoporosis, because bones naturally become less dense and weaker as you age.	**MODIFIED** This applies far less in many Asian and African countries, where people follow their traditional diet and lifestyle.

Body size and shape	Small-framed, thin-boned women are considered to be at greater risk. Women in the lowest 25% of the population for body weight are considered to be at increased risk for fracture, while women who gained weight after age 25 are considered to be at lower risk of fracture.[18] Body size is also considered to be an important factor in hip-fracture risk, with fractures being more than twice as likely in women 1.73 m (5 ft 8 in) or taller than in women 1.57 m (5 ft 2 in) or shorter.[19] The corresponding heights for men are 1.83 m (6 ft) and 1.75 m m (5 ft 9 in).[20]	**CHALLENGED** This appears to apply mainly to Caucasian women. Many Oriental people are very small-framed and thin-boned and, in their own countries, living their traditional life style, suffer far less osteoporosis. Many African women, too, can be small-boned or very tall and, in their own countries, living their traditional lifestyle, suffer far less osteoporosis than African Americans.
Ethnicity	In the USA, Caucasian and Asian women are statistically at highest risk. African–American and Latino women have a lower but significant risk.	**As above**
Family history	Susceptibility to fracture may be, in part, hereditary. People whose parents have a history of fractures also seem to have reduced bone mass and may be at risk for fractures. A history of fracture, including even traumatic fractures before menopause but especially low-impact fractures after menopause, substantially increases risk.[21] A family history of fragility fractures (i.e. fractures caused by a fall from a standing height or less) is a significant contributor to future fracture risk. Given the scant attention paid to osteoporosis until recently, this information is often missing from or is incorrect in a patient's medical records.	**As above**

DIET AND LIFESTYLE FACTORS

A lifetime diet low in calcium

STRONGLY CHALLENGED WHO confirms that countries with low intakes of calcium do not have increased osteoporosis.[22] See especially Chapters 3 and 7.

A lifetime diet low in vitamin D

MODIFIED See Chapter 6, Lifestyle Factor 1.

An inactive lifestyle or extended bed rest

CHALLENGED Bones remineralise even in astronauts after extended periods of weightlessness.

Cigarette smoking

MODIFIED

Excessive use of alcohol

MODIFIED

Ingestion of caffeine
(from coffee or chocolate, for example)

AGREED AND EXPANDED

Excessive sodium intake (from adding lots of salt to food, for example), which promotes increased excretion of calcium via the kidneys.

AGREED

MEDICAL CONDITIONS

Hormone excess produced by disease of the parathyroid, thyroid or adrenal glands.

AGREED

Hormone deficiency
● especially low oestrogen levels in women (after the menopause, especially premature menopause) and abnormal absence of menstrual periods (including because of excessive exercise in women athletes).

MODIFIED IN PART

● low testosterone levels in men (including as a result of removal of the testes to control some types of advanced cancer).	**AGREED**
● deficiency of some pituitary hormones, including prolactin, caused by tumours or underactivity of the pituitary gland – the master gland of the body, located close to the base of the skull.	**AGREED**
Eating disorders such as anorexia and bulimia	**AGREED**, but bone can be remineralised if the condition can be overcome.
Miscellaneous including: gastrectomy (removal of stomach); kidney disease.	**AGREED**
Idiopathic hypercalciuria (a frightening-sounding condition – which simply means too much calcium in the urine, of unknown cause!).	**MEANINGLESS JARGON**
Paraplegia, quadriplegia	**AGREED** unless appropriate physiotherapy is used. See also Chapter 6, Lifestyle Factor 6.

DOCTOR-INDUCED OSTEOPOROSIS

(Doctor-induced illnesses of all types are disguised from the rest of us by the use of the term iatrogenic – from the Greek iatros, meaning physician.) The following medications are of concern if not properly monitored and controlled, especially if prescribed over the long term.

Thyroxine	Used for the long-term treatment of an underactive thyroid gland. Can cause problems with bone mass.	**AGREED**
Heparin	Used to prevent blood clotting, especially during pregnancy.	Could be helped by changing to the Plant Programme diet

Warfarin	Used to reduce the risk of blood clotting in patients at high risk of stroke or heart disease.	**AS ABOVE**
Cyclosporine	Used as an immunosuppressant, e.g. in organ transplantation.	**AGREED**
Glucocorticoids (including cortisol or hydrocortizone	Medications prescribed for a wide range of disease, including arthritis, asthma, eczema, lupus, Crohn's disease and other diseases of the lungs, kidneys and liver. Experience with inhaled corticosteroids used in the treatment of asthma has not yet confirmed that they are less detrimental to the skeleton than other corticosteroids, but initial studies suggest that this might be the case.[23]	Where possible, find out the fundamental cause (especially for allergic conditions) and try to eliminate it rather than just treating symptoms (see Chapter 6, Lifestyle Factor 3)
Certain antiseizure drugs, such as phenytoin and barbiturates		**AGREED**
Gonadotropin-releasing hormone (GnRH) analogs	Used to treat endometriosis.	**AGREED**
Aluminum-containing antacids if used in excess	Used to treat stomach acidity.	Where possible find out fundamental cause of excess acidity, bearing in mind that the stomach is meant to be a bag of extremely strong acid

		(see Chapter 2, and also Chapter 6, Lifestyle Factor 1)
Certain other cancer treatments		**AGREED** but bones can remineralise.
Aromatase inhibitors	There is some concern about the potential long-term effects of using such highly effective oestrogen-depriving agents, especially on how they will affect bone integrity in post-menopausal women.[24]	**AGREED** but bones can remineralise, depending on dose and length of use.

It has also been suggested that doctor-induced hip fractures sometimes occur, and the risk increases with use of long-acting tranquillisers known as benzodiazepines.[25] Recent studies suggest that use of long-acting contraceptives, such as medroxy-progesterone acetate, may limit skeletal growth during puberty, but this observation requires confirmation.[26] Also Lee[27] raises concerns about diuretics and antibiotics. He claims that several diuretics increase urinary excretion of minerals, including calcium, while others retain calcium but may increase fracture risk by causing nocturnal urination which, among the elderly, increases the risk of accidental falls in the bathroom. In the case of antibiotics his concern centres on the use of long-term or frequent courses of broad-spectrum antibiotics that kill friendly intestinal bacteria that make vitamin K for us. Vitamin K is an important bone-building vitamin.

It is important to discuss the use of any of these drugs with your physician if you are concerned about developing osteoporosis, but you should certainly not stop or alter your medication dose on your own.

It is acknowledged[28] that some people with osteoporosis have several of these risk factors while others who develop the disease have none. Joanne, Mary and Harriet and most of the many other sufferers that we know have hardly had a day's illness in their lives, other than typical childhood diseases, before being diagnosed with osteoporosis. None has used any of the bone-damaging medications for acute health problems, let alone long-term treatment. None of them has smoked – except, some of them, for a short period when they were younger. They do not drink to excess – no more than a few glasses of wine with a meal. They all eat what most experts on osteoporosis would consider to be a healthy diet, containing a high proportion of dairy produce as a source of calcium and they take calcium and vitamin D and other mineral supplements. They are all active women, many of them taking regular exercise, and they include several golf and skiing enthusiasts.

Just as in Jane's case when, after her initial diagnosis of breast cancer, her hospital's questionnaire established that according to established risk factors she was at low risk of developing the disease, the women we have talked to would all be at low risk of developing osteoporosis based on the established risk factors listed above. Could it be that, as Jane has suggested in the case of breast cancer,[29] some of the risk factors might simply translate into indicators of a Western middle-class lifestyle and not mean much in themselves, while others are wrong or misleading?

As Earth scientists, we are both trained to piece together isolated observations and facts to develop hypotheses about natural phenomena. Hypotheses developed in this way are usually accepted and established only when they can be used to predict outcomes in similar situations. Let us give you a couple of examples that illustrate how observational science is so different from experimental science:

In the second half of the nineteenth century there was a tremendous argument raging about the age and evolution of the Earth. Natural scientists such as Charles Lyell and the famous Charles Darwin suggested, on the basis of careful and extensive observation of rocks and fossils, that the Earth and its life forms had required more than 3,000 million years to evolve to where they are today. At the time, these views were vehemently opposed by other scientists, including the famous physicist, Lord Kelvin. Kelvin used thermodynamics (a more mathematical branch of science, and therefore generally considered to be more rigorous) to calculate that a sphere of the size and composition of the Earth would have taken only 20 million years to cool to its present state from a near molten condition. Brilliant mathematics, but Kelvin's work failed to take account of the internal heat generated by the Earth's natural radioactivity. There was a very good reason for this – the Earth's natural radioactivity was not discovered until 1896 (by the French scientist Henri Becquerel). Now scientists are able to use the latest analytical techniques on a meteorite formed at the same time as the Earth to calculate that the Earth is about 4,500 million years old. This result is consistent with all other observed and measured geological evidence, and confirms that those amazing natural scientists, Lyell and Darwin, were right. Kelvin's calculation was wrong by a factor of 225 – an amazing mistake for a physicist! Score: observational scientists – 1; experimental and theoretical scientists – 0!

Another situation in which observational science proved to be far more effective than mathematical or experimentally based science occurred during the Second World War. According to Lord Dalton,[30] at the time when British shipping was being devastated by German U-boats in the early years of the war, mathematicians were employed to try to predict the distribution and courses of the U-boats. Despite their careful calculations, they had a very high failure rate. Chemists and physicists were then brought in, but they also failed in the task. Apparently it was not until geologists, who are spatially oriented scientists, skilled at integrating and predicting from very patchy or isolated observations in three dimensions, were called in that any useful predictions were made.

The medical equivalent of this type of observational science is epidemiology, which began literally as the study of epidemics in the mid-nineteenth century. At that time, Dr John Snow made his famous dot map of cholera deaths in relation to water pump distribution during the epidemic in London in 1854. He observed that the deaths occurred almost entirely among those using a water pump in Broad Street. He had the pump handle removed, and so ended the epidemic that had taken more than five hundred lives.

In a radio interview, Professor Sir Richard Doll, one of the greatest and most famous epidemiologists, recently discussed his ground-breaking work, which, some fifty years ago, established the link between lung cancer and smoking tobacco. In the radio interview, Professor Doll described how he knew he was right when he began to realise that he could predict whether a patient suffering from lung disease would be diagnosed with lung cancer or not, based on their history of tobacco smoking. Even though we do not know to this day which of the many chemical carcinogens in tobacco smoke causes lung cancer, it is firmly established that stopping smoking completely (or, ideally, never smoking at all) greatly reduces the incidence of lung cancer.[31] There are other causes of lung cancer but, in the UK alone, identifying the link between lung cancer and smoking has led to many people giving up the habit, approximately halving the death rate from the disease.[32]

What we are looking for is a means by which doctors can remove the pump handle, or a way to identify a factor or factors that people themselves can use to change their behaviour and cut the dreadful toll of osteoporosis.

DIAGNOSIS, PREVENTION AND TREATMENT

Let us look now at what happened to Joanne, Mary and Harriet, beginning with the diagnosis of their disease. Joanne, you will recall, had suffered a hip fracture, which is one of the most traumatic results of osteoporosis because it results in sudden immobility. The hip is particularly susceptible to osteoporosis, and therefore to fracture. Joanne was admitted to a National Health hospital ward specialising in osteoporosis and other bone conditions. Initial X-rays showed a fractured hip – more specifically, a fracture of the narrow neck at the top of the femur (thigh bone) before the bone widens again to form the ball that fits into the hip socket in the pelvis. This is where osteoporosis-related hip fractures usually occur. A normal X-ray of bone can identify spinal fractures and explain pain, height loss or deformity of the back, but it cannot reliably measure bone density. Joanne had a DEXA scan, which is a simple, painless procedure associated with a very small increase in the dose of ionising radiation to the body. DEXA scans require no injections, invasive procedures, sedation or any other advanced preparations, and the patient can wear light clothing. Ideally the results will be interpreted by a senior radiologist trained and

DETECTION[33]

Following a comprehensive medical assessment, your doctor may recommend that you have your bone mass measured. The most commonly used techniques include dual-energy X-ray absorptiometry (DEXA or DXA) or dual-photon absorptiometry (DPA). These methods depend on the energy from an X-ray or photon beam being deflected or absorbed when it strikes the minerals that make up bones and enable soft tissue absorption to be corrected for. The greater the mineral density, the greater the loss of beam energy. This is calculated by computer and compared with the WHO average (page 5) in order to calculate your score. A DEXA scan of the hip gives an x-ray dose similar to a chest x-ray. Other diagnostic techniques include quantified CT scan (QCT) and, more recently, ultrasound methods. Other methods include single-energy X-ray absorptiometry (SXA) and radiographic absorptiometry (RA). QCT is the most accurate bone mineral density test, and ultrasound the least accurate. QCT, however, is not widely available and the radiation dose is higher than using DEXA.[34] Some bone mineral density tests measure bone density in the spine, wrist, and/or hip (the most common sites of fractures due to osteoporosis), while others measure the density of bone in the heel or hand. It should be remembered, however, that changes in bone mineral density in the heel may show up later than those in the lower back or hip. All of these tests are painless, non-invasive and generally considered safe. Bone density tests can:

● Detect low bone density before a fracture occurs
● Confirm a diagnosis of osteoporosis if you already have a fracture
● Predict your chances of sustaining a fracture in the future, and of particular value
● Determine your rate of bone loss and/or monitor the effects of treatment if the test is conducted at intervals of a year or more

Each technique for measuring bone density measures different bone characteristics and hence may give different results. Even machines based on the same principle of measurement may give somewhat different results because, like all analytical machines, they are slightly different and may not have been adequately calibrated and standardised against each other. This is particularly important where serial measurements are made to monitor rates of bone loss or improvements in bone mineral density. See also the concerns raised on pages 4–5 about the value of individual bone mineral density measurements.

experienced in interpreting such scans. The procedure involved Joanne lying down on the machine for a few minutes with her legs elevated while an X-ray arm passed over her to prepare an image of her hip and spine. Some centres have machines that measure the density of the wrist or heel using ultrasound.

Joanne asked for full information, and was told that she had a score of –3.5 and hence was suffering from osteoporosis, with particular problems in her left hip and lower back. She was given support by her family and friends during her immobility and discussed medication fully and carefully with her specialist and family doctor. She takes a low dose of a bisphosphonate-type drug, and regularly follows a sensible exercise plan worked out for her by her physiotherapist. But she also follows the diet and supplement regimen described in Chapters 5 and 6. (Indeed, Jane included advice on the treatment of osteoporosis in *Your Life in Your Hands* because she researched the subject for Joanne at the time of her diagnosis.) She has had no further problems. Her bone mineral density has improved greatly, and her blood chemistry has been declared 'normal'. When her doctors express surprise at her progress, Joanne tries to tell them about her diet and lifestyle. Apparently they look very bemused and say that if she finds it helpful and it helps her to think positively that is fine, but they express no further interest. Being married to a scientist and knowing lots of other scientists she finds this strange, but few clinical doctors have the time or resources to follow up such information or carry out their own research. Hence there is a growing gulf in understanding between clinical doctors at the coalface and those carrying out research aimed at developing new drugs or treatments.

Mary's experience has been much worse than Joanne's. She could not accept the diagnosis, and in the following weeks she paid to see at least two more specialists privately. She had two further scans and each one gave different results, although unfortunately she did not write them down, and could not remember the scores. Also, she had different advice on the best medication regimen to follow. Eventually she settled down to attending the clinic of one specialist and began taking hormone replacement therapy. She attends a private gym, where she pays for a personal trainer. She follows, to the letter, the advice on diet and lifestyle given to her by her doctor. Sadly, her condition has deteriorated – most noticeably in the curvature of her spine and her height loss of about two inches.

Harriet's story is very similar to Mary's, although with her medical connections she has followed a far more consistent approach. Sadly her condition is much worse than Joanne's or Mary's. She now walks with two sticks, has lost much height, and even her face appears somewhat misshapen. Like Mary, Harriet kept very strictly to the dietary and lifestyle measures suggested by her doctors. These are closely similar to the standard advice

---

MEDICATIONS[35]

The drugs most commonly used against osteoporosis include:

● Bisphosphonates (also termed diphosphonates), which work by inhibiting and promoting cell-suicide of osteoclasts (see Chapter 2) and they indirectly stimulate osteoblasts. They are given orally and are poorly absorbed, especially in the presence of food – particularly milk. About 50% of the dose accumulates at sites of bone mineralisation where it can remain for months or years. Unwanted effects include gastrointestinal upsets and occasionally bone pain. According to Lee,[36] these drugs inhibit resorption of old bone, leading to a rise in bone mineral density, even though the older, 'preserved' bone will have less tensile strength.

● Oestrogens, especially for post-menopausal women. This is discussed elsewhere in this chapter (pages 21 and 22) and also in Chapter 6 (pages 112–16).

● Antioestrogens, such as tamoxifen, which have oestrogenic effects on bone.

● Vitamin D and parathyroid hormone (PTH). Vitamin D is usually given orally, but excessive intakes, including as a result of self-administration, can cause constipation, depression, weakness, fatigue, kidney stones and, in serious situations, kidney failure. PTH is being clinically trialled for the treatment of osteoporosis.

● Calcitonin, which is given by injection. Unwanted effects include nausea and vomiting, a tingling sensation in the hands, and facial flushing.

● Calcium salts. Often given with oestrogen for post-menopausal osteoporosis and vitamin D for some types of medication-induced osteoporosis. Unwanted effects include gastrointestinal disturbances. (See Chapter 6, Lifestyle Factor 1.)

given by the US National Institute of Health, Osteoporosis,[37] the Osteoporosis Society of Canada[38] and the National Osteoporosis Society in the UK.[39] Now, let us look at this standard advice in more detail:

PREVENTION

To reach optimal peak bone mass and continue building new bone tissue as you get older, there are several factors you should consider:

CALCIUM

**WE CHALLENGE MOST OF THIS ADVICE –
SEE CHAPTERS 3, 4 AND 7**

An inadequate supply of calcium over the lifetime is thought to play a significant role in contributing to the development of osteoporosis. Many published studies show that low calcium intakes appear to be associated with low bone mass, rapid bone loss, and high fracture rates. National nutrition surveys in America have shown that many people consume less than half the amount of calcium recommended (see Table 1.1) to build and maintain healthy bones. Good sources of calcium include low-fat dairy products, such as milk, yoghurt, cheese and ice cream; dark green, leafy vegetables, such as broccoli, collard greens, bok choy and spinach; sardines and salmon with bones; tofu; almonds; and foods fortified with calcium, such as orange juice, cereals and breads. Depending upon how much calcium you get each day from food, you may need to take a calcium supplement. The body's need for calcium changes during one's lifetime. Demand for calcium is greater during childhood and adolescence, when the skeleton is growing rapidly, and during pregnancy and breastfeeding. Post-menopausal women and older men also need to consume more calcium. This may be caused by inadequate amounts of vitamin D, which is necessary for intestinal absorption of calcium. Also, as you age, your body becomes less efficient at absorbing calcium and other nutrients. Older adults also are more likely to have chronic medical problems and to use medications that may impair calcium absorption.

Table 1.1 **RECOMMENDED CALCIUM INTAKES (mg/DAY)**[40]

National Academy of Sciences (1997)		National Institutes of Health (1994)	
Age		**Age**	
Birth to 6 months	210	Birth to 6 months	400
6 months to 1 year	270	6 months to 1 year	600
1–3	500	1–10	800–1200
4–8	800	11–24	1200–1500
9–13	1300	25–50 (women & men)	1000
14–18	1300	51–64 (women on ERT	1000
19–30	1000	& men)	
31–50	1000	51+ (women not on ERT)	1500
51–70	1200	65 or older	1500
70 or older	1200		
Pregnant or lactating	1000	Pregnant or lactating	1200–1500
14–18	1300		
19–50	1000		

The National Academy data are from a report[41] from the US Institute of Medicine, aimed at decreasing the risk of chronic disease through good nutrition. The first of a series of reports on Dietary Reference Intakes (DRIs) reviews calcium, phosphorus, magnesium, vitamin D, and fluoride, which are considered to be related to the health of bones.[42] The reports update and expand the Recommended Dietary Allowances (RDAs) set by the National Academy of Sciences since 1941.

VITAMIN D
MODIFIED – CHAPTER 6, LIFESTYLE FACTOR 1

Vitamin D plays an important role in calcium absorption and in bone health. It is synthesised in the skin through exposure to sunlight. While many people are able to obtain enough vitamin D naturally, studies show that vitamin D production decreases in the elderly, in people who are housebound, and during the winter. These individuals may require vitamin D supplementation to ensure a daily intake of between 400 and 800 IU of vitamin D. Large doses are not recommended.

EXERCISE
MODIFIED AND EXTENDED – CHAPTER 6, LIFESTYLE FACTOR 6

Like muscle, bone is living tissue that responds to exercise by becoming stronger. The best exercise for your bones is weight-bearing exercise, which forces you to work against gravity. These exercises include walking, hiking, jogging, stair-climbing, weight training, tennis, and dancing. Exercise not only improves your bone health, but it increases muscle strength, co-ordination, and balance and leads to better overall health. While exercise is good for someone with osteoporosis, it should not put any sudden or excessive strain on your bones. As extra insurance against fractures, your doctor can recommend specific exercises to strengthen and support your back.

SMOKING
MODIFIED AND EXTENDED – CHAPTER 6, LIFESTYLE FACTOR 8

Smoking is bad for your bones as well as for your heart and lungs. Women who smoke have lower levels of oestrogen than non-smokers and frequently go through menopause earlier. Post-menopausal women who smoke may require higher doses of hormone replacement therapy and may have more side effects. Smokers also may absorb less calcium from their diets.

ALCOHOL
MODIFIED AND EXTENDED – CHAPTER 6, LIFESTYLE FACTOR 4

Regular consumption of 60 to 90 ml, or 2 to 3 ounces a day of alcohol may be damaging to the skeleton, even in young women and men (90 ml of alcohol is a whole bottle of wine). Those who drink heavily are more prone to bone loss and fractures, both because of poor nutrition and because of increased risk of falling.

TREATMENT
MODIFIED AND EXTENDED – CHAPTERS 3, 4, 5 AND 6

A comprehensive osteoporosis treatment programme includes a

focus on proper nutrition, exercise, and safety issues to prevent falls that may result in fractures. In addition, your physician may prescribe a medication to slow or stop bone loss, increase bone density, and reduce fracture risk.

NUTRITION
CHALLENGED – CHAPTERS 3, 4 AND 5

The foods we eat contain a variety of vitamins, minerals, and other important nutrients that help keep our bodies healthy. All of these nutrients are needed in a balanced proportion. In particular, calcium and vitamin D are needed for strong bones as well as for your heart, muscles, and nerves to function properly.

OESTROGEN
MODIFIED – CHAPTER 6, LIFESTYLE FACTOR 5

Before the menopause, women are protected by their levels of the hormone oestrogen, which both inhibits the uptake of calcium *into* the bones[43, 44, 45, 46, 47] and its removal *from* the bones. After the menopause, however, oestrogen levels are very much lower, so the bones are more vulnerable to change. As well as inhibiting uptake of calcium, oestrogen prevents the death of osteoblasts[48, 49] (the cells responsible for bone formation; see Chapter 2). Physicians now recognise the importance of using oestrogen in situations where women have low or deficient levels of oestrogen. If used early enough, this can prevent a woman's bones from becoming osteoporotic. In cases where women have low bone density or have already had fractures, oestrogen can stabilise or even improve bone density. Oestrogen replacement therapy (spelled estrogen replacement therapy in America, hence 'ERT') has been shown to reduce bone loss, increase bone density in both the spine and hip, and reduce the risk of hip and spinal fractures in post-menopausal women. In women who receive oestrogen early in menopause and continue with it for six to nine years, their overall risk of fracture is reduced by 50 per cent. ERT is administered most commonly in the form of a pill or skin patch and is effective even when started after age seventy. Experts recommend ERT for women at high risk of osteoporosis. ERT is approved for both the prevention and treatment of osteoporosis. ERT is especially recommended for women whose ovaries were removed before age fifty. Oestrogen replacement should also be considered by women who have experienced natural menopause and have multiple osteoporosis risk factors, such as early menopause, family history of osteoporosis, or below normal bone mass for their age. As with all drugs, the decision to use oestrogen should be made after discussing the benefits and risks and your own situation with your doctor.

When oestrogen is taken alone, it can increase a woman's risk of developing cancer of the uterine lining (endometrial cancer). Until recently it was thought that this risk could be eliminated by using a synthetic hormone, progestin, in combination with oestrogen (hormone replacement therapy or HRT) for those women who have not had a hysterectomy. HRT relieves menopause symptoms and has been shown to have beneficial effects on the skeleton. This is not without risks, however. Potential side effects include a fourfold increased risk of breast cancer[50] and treble the risk of cervical cancer.[51] A recent trial of oestrogen plus progestin vs. placebo was stopped, after only about 5 years of follow-up, because the results for invasive breast cancer (26 per cent increase after five years) and other serious diseases showed that the risks of the treatment exceeded the benefits.[52]

Note the great emphasis placed, in this and other similar sources of information, on the need to maintain an adequate supply of calcium throughout life: the lack of this mineral is promoted as one of the most significant contributions to the development of osteoporosis. Nutritional surveys in the USA are used to show that many people consume too little calcium (see page 18, quoted from the NIH website[53]), with advice to eat dairy produce such as cheese, yoghurt, milk and ice cream; to have food fortified with calcium, including orange juice, cereals and bread; and to take a calcium supplement. Calcium supplements are another commonly promulgated remedy.

According to many orthodox practitioners, calcium lost from the bones cannot be replaced. Several recent studies suggest, however, that, in some circumstances and given the right conditions, the body will heal itself and restore bone density. For example, studies have shown that there is a significant increase in the bone density of the hip and lower back one year after removal of parathyroid glands in patients with overproduction of parathyroid hormone (which causes calcium to be removed from the bones).[54] Research on astronauts also provides strong evidence that bone can be remineralised. Hence, during space missions, weightlessness causes a massive loss of bone mineral density but this is recovered after the astronaut's return to Earth and to normal activity. Other evidence, however, suggests that osteoporosis can reach a stage where all that can be achieved is to prevent further degeneration.

Conventional medicine also places great emphasis on vitamin D deficiency, which is receiving a great deal of attention,[55] even in the healthy elderly in the United States. A prospective, controlled study in France[56] showed that daily supplementation with 100 mg of calcium and 800 IU of vitamin D significantly decreased the incidence of hip fracture in a nursing home population. Whether this occurs through an effect on bone mineral density, or because of the known beneficial effects of vitamin D on striated muscle, was not established. The investigators did demonstrate, however, that the supplements corrected mild hyperparathyroidism (see Chapters 2 and 3).

Other studies[57, 58] have shown that a high rate of bone turnover may be associated with an increased hip-fracture risk independent of bone mineral density. The effects of high bone turnover and low bone mineral density were additive in terms of risk of fracture. Thus, one conventional medical view is that it might be cost-effective to provide 1,000 mg of calcium and 800 IU of vitamin D daily to everyone in the United States aged 75 or older.[59] For advice on vitamin D supplementation, see Chapter 6, Lifestyle Factor 1.

Note also the conventional medical advice to women to take HRT to prevent post-menopausal bone loss.

So far in this chapter we have described the advice on the prevention, diagnosis and treatment of osteoporosis that you are likely to be given by orthodox medical professionals. What is apparent from reading and hearing of the health outcomes of such treatment is that it appears to be relatively unsuccessful and in some cases, like the use of ERT/HRT, to have potentially dangerous side effects. Nevertheless, we strongly recommend that you involve your orthodox health professionals in managing the condition.

YOU AND YOUR DOCTOR

Let us try to establish some dos and don'ts for working with conventional doctors. Let us first remind you that most clinical doctors do not have a background as scientific researchers. They are mostly professional human biologists who follow a strict code of ethical and medical behaviour: the Hippocratic Oath, named after Hippocrates the ancient Greek founder of modern Western medicine. Partly as a result of litigation, medical professionals increasingly rely on the results of 'evidence-based' studies. This generally means the result of double-blind trials. These involve giving an active drug in a pure, standardised dose to one group of individuals, while another group closely matched for age, socio-economic and other factors, are given a dummy tablet, termed a placebo. Such trials are carried out in a way that neither the patient nor the doctor knows which patient is being given which pill. The results of such studies are subsequently assessed statistically by the researchers, and only if the active drug is shown to have statistically significantly better outcomes than the placebo will it be prescribed.

When you are diagnosed with a potentially long-term degenerative disease such as osteoporosis, your relationship with your GP and specialist (in the case of osteoporosis, normally a rheumatologist or orthopaedic doctor) is crucial to the outcome of your disease. It is important that you establish a good relationship with all your health professionals. Although it is only natural to be anxious and afraid, try to show your doctors that you will work with them to recover your health and that you wish to be fully involved in decisions. How can you tell whether it will be possible for you to work with your doctors in this way? Here's a quick and easy ready reckoner – it makes no claim to be scientific, but it will help you identify in your own mind the most important attributes to look for in your doctors:

A CHECK-UP FOR YOUR DOCTOR

✔ Possesses lots of common sense and explains things clearly and effectively.
✖ *Treats you arrogantly or impatiently and falls back on confusing jargon if questioned.*

✔ Follows his or her chosen vocation because s/he obviously cares about people.
✖ *Authoritarian – gets a kick out of telling you what to do, gets angry when you ask questions or suggest what is wrong with you.*

✔ Demonstrates s/he is up to date in their knowledge.
✖ *Indicates s/he is ignorant of subjects that they should understand. Dismisses information, even from the peer-reviewed scientific literature.*

✔ Technically skilful, e.g. knows how to carry out a thorough physical examination.
✖ *Fails to give thorough examination or to come up with a meaningful diagnosis.*

✔ Prepared to discuss your health with you on a partnership basis and to recommend dietary, lifestyle or other factors you can change yourself.
✖ *Uninterested in underlying cause and displays a clear preference for empirical (suck it and see) methods to suppress symptoms; reaches for the prescription pad or computer keyboard before you have started your second sentence. Believes giving advice is a matter for nurses.*

A frequent problem that patients encounter is the use by the medical profession of language which seems calculated to be obscure. In fact, more than two thousand years ago the Greek physician Hippocrates warned doctors, 'Those things which are sacred are to be imparted only to sacred persons; and it is not lawful to impart them to the profane until they have been initiated in the mysteries of the science.' Today, too many doctors still seem to be following this advice. Before a medical student can become a doctor, s/he must be initiated into the secrets of a language which, it has been estimated, contains 10,000 new words – words which, to most of us, seem just as extinct as the Greek or Latin from which they originated.[60] Remember (page 9 above) that some doctors will tell you grandly that you are suffering from idiopathic hypercalciuria, instead of simply telling you that you have too much calcium in your urine and they do not know why. Always insist on fully understanding what your doctor is saying to you, and if s/he starts to use new and alarming-sounding words, make sure you ask them to explain precisely what they are trying to tell you in simpler language. Once you understand the language your doctor is using, clarify any details by asking that they draw you a diagram, for instance. Then you will be in a much stronger position to evaluate, influence and, if necessary, query your diagnosis and treatment.

CONVENTIONAL MEDICINE: SOME DOS AND DON'TS

● Especially during and after menopause, measure your weight and height and note any marked changes not explained by increased fat or muscle as a result of exercising or dieting. Also watch out for any marked unexplained changes in your shape. If friends make any comment suggesting that they have noticed some change in you, check out their observation.

● If you belong to a large general medical practice and have particular concerns about osteoporosis you might want to ask if any of the partners has any particular expertise or interest in the condition and if so ask to be referred or transferred to their care. Good health centres increasingly provide such information on their websites.

● If you are prescribed any of the medications listed on pages 9–11, especially if you are likely to need them for a long time, discuss the possible future impact on your bones with your doctor.

● If you or any of your family have a history of fractures or osteoporosis (including under its old name of 'brittle bone disease') ensure that you make your medical professionals aware. It may well be in your notes but often such information is difficult to find in the short time available for most consultations.

● If you notice any marked change or have pain in bones or joints, particularly if you are over fifty or otherwise at risk, seek medical attention.

● If your GP considers it necessary to refer you to a consultant for specialist advice – normally a rheumatologist or an orthopaedic doctor – ask him/her to recommend a good specialist, even if you intend to seek private treatment.

● Attend for all the tests and follow instructions closely.

● Ask that the same scanning machine is used (otherwise it is difficult and sometimes impossible to measure positive or negative changes in bone mineral density).

● If you pay for a private scan, check that the results will be interpreted and reported by an expert radiologist.

● Do not do what Mary did. Do not rush around in a panic from one expert to another; they may well be using different machines giving different results for bone mineral density. Find someone you trust to work with and establish a partnership to work towards regaining your health.

● Some laboratories that can be found on the internet offer urine tests for the waste products of osteoclasts – the cells that break down bones. It is claimed that there will be high levels of such substances in urine if bone is being broken down faster than it is being replaced. Consult your general medical practitioner before paying for such a test and if you decide to go ahead involve him or her in discussing the results.

● Some clinics also offer ultrasound tests of the heel bone. Again, talk to your doctor before paying for such tests and if you decide to have the test involve them in discussing the results and their implications.

● If you decide to follow our diet and lifestyle, do not expect your conventional doctors or specialists to understand immediately, but do ask them to review the evidence, including the scientific publications on which our recommendations are based.

● We always use our conventional physicians as specialists in conventional medicine, but nevertheless discuss with them any dietary or other lifestyle changes we make to complement their treatment.

● Involve your friends and family in supporting you.

● Try not to think of bad scenarios. Focus on all the things you will do when your bone health improves.

A FINAL THOUGHT

Modern medicine teaches that pain means sickness. It does not recognise that pain is also the body's way of informing us that we are doing something wrong. Pain can tell us that we are smoking too much, eating too much, or eating the wrong things.[61]

KEY POINTS

● Osteoporosis is a disease characterised by low bone mass and deterioration of bone tissue leading to increased fragility and risk of fracture particularly of the hip, spine and wrist. It has been called the 'silent disease' because initially it may be without symptoms.

● The orthodox risk factors are gender, age, body size and shape, ethnicity, family history, and certain diet and lifestyle factors, but we challenge many of these.

● Many prescribed and over-the-counter medications such as antacids can be associated with increased risk of osteoporosis, especially if used over the long term.

● Several of the medicines used by orthodox doctors to treat osteoporosis can have serious side effects.

● Work with your doctor and discuss with them the dietary and lifestyle changes we recommend, bearing in mind they are likely for legal and professional reasons to keep to their traditional treatments.

2 Bare Bones and Bags of Water

Before setting off on our scientific detective story we need to be well equipped. As Sherlock Holmes would have told Dr Watson, what we need first is to assemble the facts. This chapter describes some of the facts about the vital roles that the skeleton plays. These range from giving us our shape and keeping us upright and mobile to balancing our body chemistry. When we eat or do things that would change us from being essentially bags of water to bags of acid, it is our bones that provide vital alkaline minerals and bases to enable our bodies to continue to function properly.

THE ROLE OF THE BONES

Before we consider osteoporosis further and try to understand why it is now so prevalent, and why it affects some people and not others, we need to understand more fully the roles of our bones and skeleton.

A LIVING FRAMEWORK

Most of us think of skeletons as rigid, dead structures – inert things that hang in medical students' rooms or are found in archaeological digs. In fact our bones are living, growing tissues just like the liver or lungs or any other organ of the body. Bone, like all human tissue, is made of various types of cells, well supplied with blood vessels and with nerves and pain receptors. Bone also contains marrow, in which new blood cells are made.

The human skeleton is a unique structure, which comprises more than 200 bones, each with a distinct shape that reflects its function. The skeleton has several vital functions. It is the principal structural support for the muscles, enabling us to stand upright and move about. It is also protective against outside forces caused by falls or bangs for example and those generated by our own muscles.

The physical characteristics of the human skeleton are extraordinary and healthy bones are both strong and flexible. Much of bone is made of fibres of collagen, a protein that provides a soft framework for the skeleton (technically called the osteoid). That soft framework is strengthened by hard crystals of a calcium mineral called hydroxyapatite, composed mostly of calcium and phosphate. The fibres and crystals form a closely integrated overlapping structure of enormous strength. The collagen fibres give bone its great tensile strength (ability to resist being pulled apart) which is similar to that of cast iron despite being only one third of its weight.[1] The hydroxyapatite crystals give bone its great compressional strength (ability to resist squashing). Just think how strong the bones are in joints of lamb or beef.

A CHEMICAL STOREHOUSE
But the skeleton has another crucial role, which is less commonly recognised and understood, even by some medical professionals. It is the body's main store of calcium and other important chemical elements, which the body can use to help maintain the all-important chemical balance in the blood and other body fluids. The calcium hydroxyapatite crystals in bone have a very special structure that makes them especially suitable to be the body's storehouse not only of calcium, but also of some other essential chemical elements,[2] including magnesium, sodium and potassium. Clearly bone formation requires an adequate supply of calcium and phosphorus, which are readily available in properly balanced diets, such as the Plant Programme.[3, 4]

Let us look in a little more detail at how our bones and skeleton work as a type of chemical bank (technically a buffer) in storing and releasing the alkaline metal minerals as necessary, using calcium as an example. Calcium concentration in blood and fluids other than those in cells is regulated very precisely. This is because calcium plays such a key role in important processes in the body, such as in the contraction of muscles, including those of the heart, in blood clotting and in transmitting nerve impulses. Only about 1 per cent of the body's total calcium is in the cells and fluids. The other 99 per cent is in the bones and teeth of the human skeleton, much of which can be made available to other tissues and fluids of the body if it is needed. At times, the amount of calcium absorbed by the body, especially when there is also a high level of vitamin D in food or from sunlight, can be up to 30 per cent more than the tiny amounts that should be present in the body fluids. At other times a similar amount of calcium can be lost rapidly – for example, into the faeces as a result of diarrhoea.

The addition or subtraction of this amount of calcium from body fluids, if it persisted, would cause serious illness. The calcium in the bones of the skeleton provides the body's first line of defence to stop this happening. The process is also helped by other tissues of the body, especially the liver and intestine. Initially bone salts such as carbonates and phosphates which lack the hard, crystalline structure of hydroxyapatite are involved in the exchange. These bone salts are especially easy to dissolve and are thus able to release calcium or other minerals stored in the skeleton into the blood stream. Equally, they are readily precipitated in the bone when body fluid levels become too high. This reaction must be rapid to prevent problems with the functioning of the heart muscles or nerves, and it is because the newly formed bone salts are very small and their surface area very large that they are able to act as such an excellent fast-acting bank.

Hence the bones serve as large reservoirs or banks, releasing calcium when extra-cellular fluid concentration falls below the precise levels needed for body functions to work properly and storing excess calcium when extra-cellular fluid concentration becomes too high. The skeleton and bones work in a similar manner to regulate levels of magnesium, phosphorus and other elements which are crucial in maintaining correct body function. More than half of the body's magnesium is stored in the bones, for example. Bone also acts to conserve phosphorus, the most important element in the energy cycle of all life forms.

A RENEWABLE STRUCTURE

Bone is continually being remodelled. Old bone is resorbed by special cells called osteoclasts, and new bone is formed by other special cells called osteoblasts. The continued deposition and absorption of bone has several important functions. The shape of the bone can be changed in response to changing stress on bone during our lives. For example, bone can readily adjust to different degrees of stress – thickening over time in individuals required to carry heavy loads. Also old bone becomes relatively brittle and weak as its organic matrix degenerates and has to be replaced by bone with a new organic matrix. Finally, remodelling ensures that bone remains strong throughout our lives and that small cracks and defects are repaired and larger fractures are healed. Here are some of the chemicals that have a role in bone remodelling.

The Role of Some Chemical Messengers in Maintaining Bone

● Parathyroid hormone (PTH), secreted by small glands near the thyroid in the neck, responds to a fall in blood calcium by stimulating osteoclasts to resorb bone. It also increases resorption of calcium by the kidney.

● Vitamin D formed by sunlight in the skin or available from foods such as oily fish (see Chapter 4) promotes bone mineralisation.

● Calcitonin, produced by special cells in the thyroid gland, has the opposite effect from PTH and depresses osteoclast activity.

● Other hormones and chemicals are involved in the process of bone remodelling, including oestrogen and progesterone in females, and testosterone in males.

● Osteogenic (bone-generating) proteins are also involved in bone remodelling in both sexes.[5] These include the growth factors erythropoietin (EPO) and insulin-like growth factor-1 (IGF-1).

The rate at which bone is remodelled is quite remarkable.[6] Dense (or cortical) bone of the shafts of long bones is tightly cast in long strands around minute tubular channels for the passage of nutrients and bone remodelling cells. The turnover time for 100 per cent renewal is about ten to twelve years. Other less dense bone – trabecular (meaning little beams) bone – forms an open meshwork of little struts and is found mostly at the end of long bones, in the heel and in vertebral bones. The 100 per cent turnover time for these bones is about four to five years. Thus osteoporosis – and recovery from osteoporosis – will show itself first in trabecular bone. In advanced osteoporosis, thinning and reduction in the number of bone trabeculae is combined with thinning of the cortical bone.

Until early adulthood, bones become larger, heavier and denser, because the process of bone formation is more important than bone resorption. Bone mass normally reaches its maximum strength and density in our mid-twenties. It then remains stable, with a balance between resorption and formation, until middle age – a few years before the menopause in women. At this time bone loss begins to outstrip bone formation, and bone loss becomes increasingly important with increasing age. All this is part of the normal process of ageing. According to orthodox medicine the rate of bone loss can accelerate tenfold during menopause or with castration in men and then settles down to 1–3 per cent a year.[7] The loss during menopause is attributed to increased osteoclast activity mainly affecting trabecular bone. The loss in both sexes in later life is attributed to decreased osteoblast numbers mainly affecting cortical bone.[8] In some people, however, bone mass is decreased below the normal range, leading to especially fragile bones at increased risk of fracture – the condition known as osteoporosis, in which bones are damaged prematurely. Osteo, from the Greek, simply means bone, and porosis, similarly, means porous, which describes how osteoporotic bones look inside. Normal bone marrow contains small holes, but osteoporotic bones have much larger holes and look spongy. In osteoporotic bone, less osteoblasts are available,[9, 10, 11, 12, 13, 14, 15, 16] and/or the activity of osteoblasts is impaired,[17, 18, 19, 20] giving rise to prematurely aged bones.[21, 22] In osteoporotic bones there is less matrix available that can be calcified than in healthy bones.[23, 24, 25] Also in osteoporosis dead cells are not replaced, and microfractures are not repaired.[26,27] Advanced osteoporosis involves bone salts, hydroxyapatite and the organic protein matrix of bone.[28] Later, in Chapters 5 and 6 and in Section 2, we shall give you advice on how to arrest and, hopefully, improve this condition but let us first try to understand the fundamental cause of the problems.

BAGS OF WATER

So far we have looked at some of the amazing bio-mechanical and bio-chemical roles that our skeleton and bones fulfil. Without them we should be just a totally non-viable floppy heap of muscles and tissue – just think how a boned turkey or chicken carcass compares with the more usual original. Our skeletons keep us properly formed, upright and mobile and in shape. They also act as a bank of minerals to keep our bodies balanced in relation to essential chemicals such as calcium and magnesium so that essential functions of our bodies, from the beating of the heart to the transmission of signals along the nervous system and in the brain, work properly. But the skeleton and bones play another vitally important role – one that is so overwhelming that it is frequently overlooked. They have an essential part in regulating how acid or alkaline the blood and body fluids become, and this is crucial to understanding osteoporosis and working out how to prevent, treat and arrest the disease. To understand the importance of this process, the first thing we need to appreciate is that as human beings we are essentially bags of water.

According to Professor Steven Rose in his wonderful book *The Chemistry of Life*,[29] it remains true that, as the biochemist-geneticist J. B. S. Haldane said, 'even the Archbishop of Canterbury is 65 per cent water'. Whoever we are, no matter how famous or eminent, we are in fact mainly large bags of water.

The composition of the human body is shown in Table 2.1. From this it is clear that the chemical elements – oxygen and hydrogen that water is composed of – make up about 75 per cent

TABLE 2.1 **THE COMPOSITION OF THE HUMAN BODY BY WEIGHT**[30]

Class	Substance	% body weight
As elements	Oxygen	65
	Carbon	18
	Hydrogen	10
	Nitrogen	3
	Calcium*	2
	Phosphorus*	1.1
	Potassium	0.35
	Sulphur	0.25
	Sodium	0.15
	Chlorine	0.15
	Magnesium*, iron, manganese, copper, iodine, cobalt, zinc	Trace elements essential for body function
	Cadmium, lead and some radioactive elements	Trace ellements that cause harm, often locked away in the bones to protect other body functions
As water and solid matter	Water	60–80
	Total solid matter	20–40

* Note that calcium, magnesium and phosphorus make up only a little more than 3 per cent of the human body by weight – and these elements are mostly in the skeleton.

of the body by weight. Water is biologically ideal as a basis for life, because many substances including nutrients, oxygen and many other chemicals essential to life can dissolve in it and be transported around the body.[31] Because water is such an excellent medium for dissolving substances, it is rarely pure in nature. Many substances when dissolved in water cause it to become either acid or alkaline. The extent to which this happens is expressed by a special type of numerical scale, representing the acidity or alkalinity of the solution, which is called the pH of the solution.

The pH of a solution is of overwhelming importance in chemistry including that of our bodies. It is one of the main controls affecting how all other chemicals behave. For those who wish to learn a little more about acids, alkalis, salts and pH to understand the implication of such factors to the development of osteoporosis please see the appendix at the end of this chapter. All we need to understand here is that acids, if they are not neutralised, are very corrosive. They actively corrode metals. Even gold, one of the least reactive metals, is attacked by a mixture of nitric and hydrochloric acids – a mixture called 'aqua regia' (royal water). Alkaline minerals such as calcium, on the other hand, neutralise acids in a neutralisation reaction. The reaction (in words) is:

acid plus alkali makes water plus a salt

KEEPING THE BALANCE

Human body chemistry continues to be based on that of ancestral organisms, and reflects the ancient alkaline ocean environment in which they evolved. Thus, our body's internal environment remains slightly alkaline, with a blood-plasma pH, ideally, of 7.4. Most of our enzymatic, immunologic and repair mechanisms all function at their best when the body and blood can maintain this pH. The body has many checks and balances to maintain its pH within a very narrow range.

A small change in pH can have a profound effect on body function. For example, the ability of muscle to contract declines, and levels of hormones like adrenaline and aldosterone increase, if the body becomes even slightly more acid. In addition, different parts of the body have different levels of acidity and alkalinity. Some of these are shown in Table 2.2.

It is clear that, while there can be a wide range of pH values for the saliva and urine, the value for the blood is maintained within very narrow bounds – the 'cleaned-up' arterial blood being slightly more alkaline than the blood that has been around the body and is being returned to the heart-lung system through the veins. The normal pH of arterial blood is 7.4,[32]

TABLE 2.2 **pH OF VARIOUS BODY TISSUES**[33, 34]

TISSUE	pH
Skeletal muscle	6.9–7.2
Heart	7.0–7.4
Liver	7.2
Brain	7.1
Blood	7.35–7.4
Saliva	6.0–7.4
Urine	4.5–8.0
Stomach	0.8–3.0

whereas the pH of venous blood is about 7.35, because of the extra amounts of carbon dioxide (CO_2) it contains (which forms carbonic acid).

While this slightly alkaline internal balance is optimal, our biochemical functioning, including many life processes, produces acid. When we exercise or move we produce lactic acid and carbon dioxide which turns into carbonic acid in water. Even breathing in a stuffy, unventilated environment can cause CO_2 levels in the body to rise, increasing the acidity of the blood. Immune responses, such as allergies and hypersensitivity, and even stress, directly and indirectly, can generate substantial amounts of acids that affect our metabolism. Cold weather acidifies the blood, whereas hot weather alkalises the blood.[35] Also, as we shall discuss later, many of the foods we eat generate acids (see Chapter 4). For the blood and body fluids to maintain the essential alkaline state, acids from all sources must be neutralised through combination with alkaline minerals and bases and, as we have learned, it is our bones and skeleton which release these as the body's first line of defence against acidosis.

According to Professor Rose[36] regulation of body pH 'is extremely important to the delicately balanced living cell where sharp fluctuations in acidity and alkalinity can easily spell disaster'. Because of the importance of the acid–alkaline balance in the blood and tissues, the body has several mechanisms, in addition to those involving the skeleton, for regulating this balance.[37, 38] Many organs in the body (especially the adrenal glands, kidneys and lungs) and other systems (e.g. haemoglobin in the blood) play important roles in maintaining a mildly alkaline, near-neutral pH in the body. But, as we shall see, diet is of immense importantce, especially over the long term.

Many body functions are involved in the regulation of acid–alkaline balance including respiration, excretion, digestion and cellular metabolism. The bloodstream also contains buffers that act chemically to resist changes in pH. Regulation of blood pH is also carried out by the lungs and kidneys. The lungs aid in acid–alkaline regulation by removing carbon dioxide from the blood. Because carbon dioxide combines with water in the body to form carbonic acid, removing carbon dioxide is equivalent to removing acid. Respiratory rates can vary depending on the acidity of the body, speeding up under acid conditions to remove carbon dioxide and reduce acidity, or slowing down under alkaline conditions to retain acid and reduce alkalinity.

The kidney also responds to the pH of the blood. If the blood is too acid, the kidney excretes extra hydrogen ions into the urine and retains extra sodium. Phosphorus in the form of phosphate is required for this exchange. The body obtains this phosphorus from bone if it is otherwise unavailable. When the bloodstream is extremely acid, the kidney uses a different method and excretes ammonium ions, each of which contains four hydrogen atoms, into the urine. When the body is too alkaline, the process is reversed, and hydrogen is retained.

In the digestive process, acid–alkaline balance is affected by the secretions of the stomach and the pancreas. These secretions are absorbed into the bloodstream and affect the rest of the body. When food is eaten, the stomach secretes hydrochloric acid. In response to this acid, the pancreas secretes bicarbonate which neutralises the stomach acid so that pancreatic enzymes can work properly. Normally, after eating, there are transient changes in blood pH, known as the acid and alkaline tides, which correspond to the stomach and pancreatic secretions. Usually the pH of the blood quickly returns to normal. However, if digestive secretions are out of balance, then the whole body can be affected. Other digestive problems that affect the body's pH are diarrhoea, which results in a loss of bicarbonate, and hence also of alkalinity, and vomiting, which results in a loss of acid.

SYMPTOMS OF OVER-ACIDITY OR OVER-ALKALINITY

Because the normal pH of arterial blood is 7.4, a person is considered to have acidosis when the pH falls below this value. When the blood is too acid, symptoms include drowsiness, which may progress to stupor and coma. Acute acidosis can result from kidney or lung problems, dehydration, ingestion of certain drugs, diabetes or diarrhoea, and is treated by giving an alkaline solution such as bicarbonate of soda.

When the pH of the arterial blood rises above 7.4 the person is considered to have alkalosis. Symptoms include cramps, muscle spasms, irritability and extreme excitability. Acute alkalosis may be caused by impaired kidney function, hyperventilation, the use of diuretic or steroid drugs, vomiting or gastric drainage. Acute alkalosis is treated by giving an acid solution, such as ammonium chloride, or by breathing expired carbon dioxide from a paper bag.[39]

The lower limit of blood pH at which a person can live for more than a few hours is 6.8, and the upper limit about 8.0.[40]

All of this is fairly well known, but what about the involvement of the bones in buffering the acid–alkaline state of our blood and body tissues? The bones, after all, contain most of the body's store of those chemicals that are the most powerful at neutralising acid, including calcium, magnesium, strontium and bicarbonate. Typical Western diets and lifestyles place demands on the role of the skeleton in buffering the acidity of the blood, and it is these demands that scientists are now suggesting is the root cause of the epidemic of osteoporosis. We shall examine the evidence in more detail in the next chapter.

KEY POINTS

● The human skeleton comprises more than 200 bones.
● Like other organs of the body such as the lungs or liver, our bones are living growing tissue, which must be renewed.
● A healthy skeleton is essential for our shape and mobility.
● Also, the skeleton is the body's main store of minerals, which it can release to neutralise acid in our blood which otherwise could cause serious damage.
● If the body is forced to do this for too long, our bones will become demineralised leading to osteoporosis.

APPENDIX

ACIDS, ALKALIS AND BASES, SALTS AND pH

We have all heard terms such as acid, alkali, base, salt and pH, either at school or because they are often used in television commercials to market products. We are told, for example, that cosmetic products are 'pH balanced' and are thus good for the skin. But what, precisely, does all this mean, and why does it matter when considering the health of our bones?

ACID PEOPLE?

When we began to study chemistry at school our teachers started the lesson on acids with a little rhyme that went something like this:

Little Johnny was a chemist
Little Johnny is no more
For what he drank as H-$_2$-O
was H-$_2$-S-O-$_4$

Many of you will know that H_2O is the chemical formula for water, and H_2SO_4 that of sulphuric acid. The point is that water is good for us – indeed we could not live without it – while acids as strong as concentrated sulphuric acid can be so powerfully corrosive that they would cause any part of the body they came into contact with, including the bones, to dissolve.

We must look at the composition of water in a little more detail. Water can be considered to be made up of hydrogen ions (H^+) and hydroxide ions (OH^-), which added together give us H_2O, in which the positive electrical charge of hydrogen ions is balanced by the negative electrical charge of hydroxide ions. It may help to think of ions as different types of tiny particles with positive and negative tags. In pure water there is a perfect balance between hydrogen ions and hydroxide ions, and water is therefore said to be neutral. If, however, there is a high proportion of hydrogen ions relative to hydroxide ions in a solution, the solution will be acid and, depending on its concentration and other factors, behave like poor little Johnny's sulphuric acid.

A high proportion of hydroxide ions in solution is not healthy either, because such solutions are strongly alkaline and are capable of attacking proteins in the body. The slippery feeling on our hands when we use strong detergents and the soreness afterwards are because of this caustic effect. Caustic soda would, in a different way, be just as bad for little Johnny as sulphuric acid.

PROPERTIES OF ACIDS[41]

Since the behaviour of acids and alkalis is so important to Johnny's health, it is worth considering some of these properties in a little more detail.

Acids turn blue litmus to red. Litmus is one of a large number of organic compounds that change colour when a solution changes from acid to alkaline at a particular point. Litmus is the oldest known pH indicator. It is red in acid solutions and blue in alkaline ones. The phrase 'litmus test' indicates that litmus has been around a long time in the English language. Litmus does not change colour exactly at the neutral point between acid and alkaline, but very close to it. Litmus is often impregnated on to paper to make 'litmus paper'.

Acids taste sour. The word 'sauer' in German means acid and is pronounced almost exactly the same way as 'sour' in English. (Sauerkraut is sour cabbage, cabbage preserved in its own fermented lactic acid.) Stomach acid is hydrochloric acid. We do not normally taste stomach acid, except as a result of vomiting, and I am sure we all remember how unpleasant and sour it tastes. Acetic acid is the acid ingredient in vinegar. Citrus fruits such as lemons, grapefruit, oranges and limes have citric acid in the juice. Sour milk, sour cream, yoghurt and cottage cheese all have lactic acid from the fermentation of the milk sugar, lactose. Vitamin C is also an acid – called ascorbic acid. Aspirin and many other non-steroidal anti-inflammatory drugs (NSAIDs), which are commonly used to treat the pain of rheumatoid and osteoarthritis, also behave as weak acids in the body.[42]

Acids (such as sulphuric and phosphoric acids) and alkalis (such as calcium hydroxide) neutralise each other by combining to make a salt and water. The hydrogen ion of the acid and the hydroxide ion of the base unite to form water.

pH AND BUFFERS

A scale based on pH values from 1 to 14 (below) is used to show how acid or alkaline a solution is. A pH of 7 is neutral, which means there is a perfect balance of hydrogen and hydroxide ions. Values less than 7 are acid, while values greater than this, up to 14, are alkaline. The scale is logarithmic, which means that for every 1.0 change in the pH value, the number of H^+ ions or OH^- ions increases tenfold. For example, a value of 6 is ten times more acid than one of 7, while a value of 5 is a hundred times more acid than one of 7, and the same applies on the alkaline scale. The table below shows that the relative variation in the number of hydrogen ions between very acid and very alkaline solutions is so great that, unless the logarithmic 1 to 14 scale is used, it is impossible to represent pH change on the same graph – or even on the same planet!

When hydrogen ions are added to a solution the pH decreases. When they are removed, or hydroxyl ions are added, the pH increases. Some substances combine with hydrogen or hydroxide and remove them from solution, thus preventing any change in pH. Such substances are called buffers. To give you some idea of the real magnitude of change we have shown the relative number of hydrogen ions for each pH value together with some examples of the pH of some body fluids (see further Table 2.2).

Relative number of hydrogen ions	The pH scale	Comments	Body fluids
1	14	very alkaline	
10	13		
100	12	alkaline	
1,000	11		
10,000	10	slightly alkaline	
100,000	9		
1,000,000	8		Blood and urine, max. (8.0)
10,000,000	7	NEUTRAL	Blood, ideal (7.35–7.4)
100,000,000	6		Blood, min. (6.8)
1,000,000,000	5		
10,000,000,000	4	slightly acid	Urine, min. (4.5)
100,000,000,000	3		Stomach, max. (3)
1,000,000,000,000	2	acid	
10,000,000,000,000	1		
100,000,000,000,000	0	very acid	Stomach, min. (0.8)

Most of the fluids in the human body (see Table 2.2) are in a narrow pH range, with the widest range in the digestive tract. For example, the stomach is a bag of hydrochloric acid with a pH as low as 0.8.[43] But note the very small ideal pH range of the blood in a normal, healthy body.

PROPERTIES OF ALKALIS[44]

Alkalis, on the other hand, release a hydroxide ion into water solution. Alkalis turn red litmus to blue. The neutralisation of sodium hydroxide (NaOH) with hydrochloric acid (HCl), for example, produces water (H_2O) and sodium chloride (NaCl, more commonly known as table salt). Salts that are dissolved in water may not be at neutral pH (7). Table salt has a neutral pH in water, but baking soda (the chemical name of which is sodium bicarbonate, or sodium hydrogen carbonate – chemical formula, $NaHCO_3$) is very alkaline when dissolved in water. Other salts, such as ammonium chloride (NH_4Cl), are acid in solution.

Alkalis denature or damage protein, which accounts for the 'slippery' feeling when your hands are exposed to some strong detergents for example. Strong alkalis, such as sodium or potassium, which dissolve well in water and form strong bases, are very dangerous, because a great amount of the structural material of the human body consists of protein. Alkalis taste bitter. Many of the most alkaline foods such as some herbs and spices taste bitter.

The terms 'alkali' and 'base' are often used synonymously. A base is an ion or molecule that can accept a hydrogen ion. The simplest example is hydroxide, OH^-, which can accept a hydrogen ion, H^+, becoming H_2O (water) in the process. An alkali is a molecule formed by a combination of one or more alkaline metals, such as sodium, potassium, calcium or magnesium, with a highly basic ion such as the hydroxyl ion, which will quickly remove hydrogen ions from solution.

Even from considering just little Johnny's plight, it is clear why the body needs to act rapidly to ensure that body fluids do not become too acid or too alkaline for any longer than is absolutely necessary. Moreover the precision with which the acidity of the blood and extracellular fluid is regulated in the body emphasises its overwhelming importance. For example, the variation in the normal hydrogen ion concentration of blood is only about one millionth that of sodium.[45]

3 Boning Up

In this chapter we explain what the peer-reviewed scientific literature has to say about the real causes of osteoporosis. We first look at the findings of studies into the incidence of osteoporotic disease in different countries. These show dramatic differences between low-incidence countries such as Nigeria and China and high-incidence countries such as the UK, USA and Germany. We then examine authoritative information on diets and other research – and find that it fails to support the suggestion that dairy consumption helps to protect against osteoporosis. Indeed the evidence is to the contrary: we find compelling evidence published by eminent American scientists that the disease is predominantly related to the Western diet. This diet contains too high a proportion of animal protein, which generates excess acid in our bodies and it is this acid that gradually leaches our bones away leading to osteoporosis.

As we saw in Chapter 1, orthodox Western medicine has traditionally viewed osteoporosis as an inevitable process associated with menopause in women and ageing in both sexes. The emphasis has been on slowing bone loss using high-calcium diets and vitamin D supplementation and other medication including HRT for post-menopausal women.[1] We shall now begin to present scientific research that indicates that we should be looking to changes in diet and lifestyle to help reverse the process. Also, rather than osteoporosis being viewed as an inevitable disease of ageing, we shall being to present evidence that with proper attention to diet and lifestyle at a young age, the disease may be largely preventable.

AROUND THE WORLD IN 33 COUNTRIES

Just as Jane showed in her book on breast cancer,[2] we can gain important clues on the cause of disease by looking at its distribution in different countries and in different communities in the world.

Because of the World Health Organisation (WHO) definition of osteoporosis as a disease of low bone density (see Chapter 1) it is difficult to find reliable information on the incidence of the disease worldwide, especially since poor countries generally have few, if any, reliable methods of measuring bone mineral density. Even if they did, it is not clear that this would be a reliable predictor of osteoporosis in non-Caucasian women. On the other hand, information on the incidence of hip fracture as a result of osteoporosis is easier to find and is generally considered to be more reliable for comparative purposes. Data on hip fracture incidence (HFI) in 'elderly' women (which is defined by researchers into osteoporosis as women over fifty years of age!) for different countries is shown in Table 3.1 and Figure 3.1 (pages 47–8). It is based on information carefully compiled and published by a team of researchers at the Department of Medicine, University of California, San Francisco.[3]

Such data must first be standardised so that we are comparing like with like, because, for example, some countries have lots of younger 'over 50s' and others lots of older people. The Californian research team have done this, carefully and rigorously, standardising to the age distribution of women in the USA in 1987 as their reference population.

The resulting data show quite dramatic differences between countries, which are rather surprising if one has been used to following the conventional wisdom on the causes of osteoporosis that we discussed in Chapter 1. Hence, in Nigeria, there is less than one hip fracture per 100,000 person years, compared with Germany and the Scandinavian countries where the HFI is up to 200 times higher. Countries with the lowest rates of HFI (less than ten) are Nigeria, China, New Guinea, Thailand and South Africa – countries that are ethnically and geographically diverse. In contrast, almost all the countries with rates higher than a hundred are similar in having a Western diet and lifestyle.

The conclusion from these data strikes you with some force. If you were living in Nigeria or China and following their traditional lifestyle your risk of suffering from osteoporosis would be one two-hundredth of that if you were living in Germany or Scandinavia and following their customary lifestyle. According to one recent

TABLE 3.1 **AGE-STANDARDISED RATES OF HIP FRACTURE INCIDENCE (HFI) IN 33 COUNTRIES***

Country	HFI per 100,000 person-years
Nigeria	0.8
China	2.9
New Guinea	3.1
Thailand	5.0
South Africa	7.7
Korea	11.5
Singapore	21.6
Malaysia	26.6
Yugoslavia	33.5
Saudi Arabia	47.3
Chile	56.8
Italy	57.2
Holland	60.7
Spain	65.1
Japan	67.3
Hong Kong	69.2
Israel	75.5
Ireland	76.0
France	77.0
Finland	93.5
Canada	110.3
Crete	113.0
United Kingdom	116.5
Portugal	119.8
United States	120.3
Australia	124.8
Switzerland	129.4
New Zealand	139.0
Argentina	147.8
Denmark	165.1
Sweden	172.0
Norway	186.7
Germany	199.3

The data are for women over the age of 50 expressed as fractures per 100,000 person-years, standardised to the age-group distribution of women in the USA in 1987

* Frassetto, L.A., Todd, K.M., Morris, R.C. Jr and Sebastian, A. 2000. Worldwide incidence of hip fracture in elderly women: relation to consumption of animal and vegetable foods. *Journal of Gerontology: Medical Sciences*, 55A, 10, M585–M592.

FIGURE 3.1 **AGE-STANDARDISED RATES OF HIP FRACTURE INCIDENCE (HFI) IN 33 COUNTRIES***

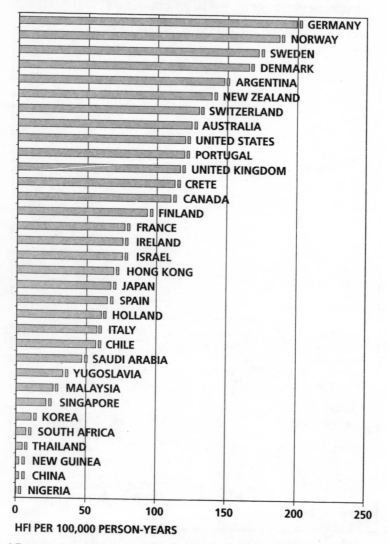

HFI PER 100,000 PERSON-YEARS

* Frassetto, L.A., Todd, K.M., Morris, R.C. Jr and Sebastian, A. 2000. Worldwide incidence of hip fracture in elderly women: relation to consumption of animal and vegetable foods. *Journal of Gerontology: Medical Sciences*, 55A, 10, M585–M592.

study,[4] an amazing 30 per cent of post-menopausal women in industrialised countries on a Western diet are osteoporotic, and this rises to 70 per cent of those aged eighty or over.

This is not because of genetic differences between black and Asian people and white people. It is clear from Table 3.1 and Figure 3.1 that there is no simple relationship between osteoporotic hip fracture incidence and ethnicity or geography. Moreover, osteoporosis incidence in female Asians living in oriental countries is much lower than in Asian females living in the USA,[5] and osteoporosis incidence (and calcium consumption) in African women[6] is much lower than in African-American women living in the USA.[7] Also, hip-fracture rates are far lower in black South Africans than in African-Americans.[8]

Just as in the case of breast cancer,[9] the data appear to suggest that some lifestyle or environmental factor is dramatically increasing the chances of developing osteoporosis for women in rich industrialised countries following a standard Western lifestyle.

SACRED COWS

We can use the data on hip fracture incidence further to examine the relevance of some of the main risk factors considered by orthodox medicine to be important in the development of osteoporotic disease. Let us examine two of these factors for which there are authoritative data on dietary intake prepared by the United Nations Food and Agriculture Organisation and published as food balance sheets:[10] first, the evidence that a diet high in calcium from dairy produce provides protection against osteoporosis, and secondly whether there is an association between alcohol consumption and osteoporotic hip fracture incidence. We will also look here at evidence that a sunny climate protects against the condition through the production of vitamin D in the skin.

CALCIUM, DAIRY, AND THE OSTEOPOROSIS CONNECTION

In Figure 3.2 we have taken the data on hip fracture incidence carefully collected and examined by Frassetto and co-workers[11] and plotted it against the average milk intake per person in each of the countries listed, using the Food and Agriculture Organisation (FAO) food balance sheets. It is quite clear that the countries with the lowest intake of whole milk consumption also have the lowest hip fracture rates. Nigeria and China, with the lowest hip-fracture rates, consume less than 10 kg of milk per person per year. Although there is considerable scatter in the diagram (which may be due to the lack of available data for total dairy products), there does appear to be some relationship between high milk consumption and high hip-fracture incidence.

There is nothing particularly new in this finding. Much other published research supports this simple result. Many Westerners consume the recommended 1000–1500 mg of calcium daily, whereas the average daily consumption in many developing countries in Africa and Asia is 500 mg of calcium or less. In these countries the intake of dairy products is low or non-existent and the incidence of osteoporosis is extremely low. According to John Robbins,[12] 'Studies comparing the bone densities of people with different diets show a pattern completely opposed to the dairy industry's declarations. The research invariably reveals greater bone resorption and development of osteoporosis with a greater intake of meat and dairy products, not the other way round.'

Here are some of the other findings that suggest that a high diary intake is associated with high rates of osteoporosis:

● Harvard University's landmark Nurses Health Study, which followed 78,000 women over a twelve-year period, found that the women who consumed the most calcium from dairy foods broke more bones than those who rarely drank milk.[13] Summarising this study, the *Lunar Osteoporosis Update* (November 1997) explained: 'This increased risk of hip fracture was associated with dairy calcium . . . If this were any agent other than milk, which has been so aggressively marketed by dairy interests, it undoubtedly would be considered a major risk factor.'

● Researchers from the University of Sydney and Westmead Hospital discovered that consumption of dairy foods, especially early in life, increases the risk of hip fractures in old age.[14]

● In Greece, the average milk consumption doubled from 1961 to 1977[15] (and was even higher in 1985), and during the period 1977–1985 the age-adjusted osteoporosis incidence also almost doubled.[16]

● In Hong Kong in 1989, twice as much dairy produce was consumed as in 1966,[17] and osteoporosis incidence tripled in the same period.[18] The milk consumption level is now almost at European levels, and so is the incidence of osteoporosis.[19] Compare this with data for China (Figure 3.1) which shows that where Chinese people live on their traditional diet they have low levels of osteoporosis-related hip fractures.

FIGURE 3.2 **RELATIONSHIP BETWEEN HIP FRACTURE INCIDENCE* AND MILK CONSUMPTION† FOR 33 COUNTRIES**

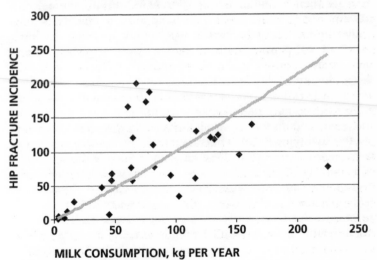

* Frassetto, L.A., Todd, K.M., Morris, R.C. Jr and Sebastian, A. 2000. Worldwide incidence of hip fracture in elderly women: relation to consumption of animal and vegetable foods. *Journal of Gerontology: Medical Sciences*, 55A, 10, M585–M592.

† *Food Balance Sheets*, 1991. Statistics Division of the Economic and Social Policy Department. Food and Agriculture Organisation of the United Nations.

● The countries where the most dairy produce is consumed include Sweden, Finland, Switzerland and The Netherlands (300 to 400 kg per person, per year), and osteoporosis incidence in these countries is high and has increased dramatically.[20, 21, 22, 23, 24, 25, 26, 27]

● Like Australians and New Zealanders,[28] Americans consume three times more milk than the Japanese, and hip-fracture incidence in Americans is 2.5 times higher.[29] Also within America, those that consume less milk, like the Mexican-Americans and African-Americans, have an osteoporosis incidence that is half that of white Americans,[30] which is not due to genetic differences.[31]

● In other countries where very little milk is consumed, for example in the Congo,[32] New Guinea[33] and Togo[34] (6 kg per person, per year) osteoporosis is extremely rare too. People do increase their bone-mineral density by consuming more calcium,[35, 36, 37, 38] and the average bone mineral density is higher in residents of countries where milk is consumed, but bone mineral density has been shown by other studies to be a poor predictor of hip and other fractures.[39, 40, 41]

● Finally, an analysis of all research conducted since 1985[42] concluded: 'If dairy food intakes confer bone health, one might expect this to have been apparent from the 57 outcomes, which included randomised, controlled trials and longitudinal cohort studies involving 645,000 person-years.' The researchers go on to express concern that 'there have been few carefully designed studies of the effects of dairy foods on bone health,' and then to conclude with typical scientific reserve that 'the body of scientific evidence appears inadequate to support a recommendation for daily intake of dairy foods to promote bone health in the general US population'.

It is worth noting also that milk contains growth factors such as IGF-1 and EPO. These so-called osteogenic proteins promote bone remodelling.[43] Could it be that their levels are increased by milk consumption, resulting in excessive bone remodelling?

Studies of osteoporosis between countries and within countries show that the less milk consumed, the lower is the osteoporosis rate.[44, 45] We think it is fair to conclude that people in countries with high hip-fracture rates generally consume more milk.

ENOUGH IS ENOUGH!

Turning to calcium, there is little evidence that, above an essential minimum, additional calcium intake will have a beneficial effect on osteoporosis and this level may be lower than that recommended by orthodox medicine (see Chapter 1), depending on other dietary factors.

For example, many of the people of Africa live on a low-protein vegetable diet. One group of African women studied take in only 350 mg of calcium per day, compared with the recommended daily allowance (RDA) of 1200 mg. They bear, on average, nine children during their lifetime and breast-feed them for two years. They do not have calcium deficiency, seldom break a bone and rarely lose a tooth.[46] They consume much less calcium than Americans, and yet are essentially free of osteoporosis,[47] whereas their genetic African-American relatives living in the USA, eating the standard American diet, have levels of osteoporosis equal to those of their white neighbours.[48]

Eskimos,[49] in contrast, have the highest dietary calcium intake of any people in the world – more than 2000 mg per day – and one of the world's highest protein intakes – 250 to 400 g per day. Despite being physically active, Eskimo people also have one of the highest rates of osteoporosis in the world.

There is even a theory that excessive calcium intake actually causes osteoporosis.[50] According to this theory, osteoporosis is about prematurely aged bones. Calcium is thought to increase bone-mineral density initially, but continued high intake may then cause the process to break down. The bones begin to look spongy and porous, and become osteoporotic. This is because osteoblasts and osteoclasts have been forced to work too hard and are essentially burned out because of forced hyperactivity.

The argument goes like this. All our organs age, because the cells in our bodies are continually wearing out – to be replaced by new ones. It is now known that the number of times the cells in the human body can renew themselves is fixed. This is determined by counting devices known as telomeres on the chromosomes. Hence if we do something that causes cells to turn over too rapidly, the affected organs will eventually age prematurely.

A good example is the effect of sunlight on our skin. If we expose our skin to the sun too much, we will look older sooner, because the sun burns the outer skin cells, which must be replaced by new cells sooner. And the sooner cells must be replaced the sooner the time comes when the skin cells cannot multiply any more. Thus, our skin appears prematurely aged.

According to this theory, more calcium is absorbed into the bones after the menopause, because of a lack of oestrogen,[51, 52, 53] stimulating the production and activity of both osteoblasts and osteoclasts.[54, 55, 56, 57, 58] As more calcium is absorbed, more is removed. Fifty to seventy per cent of the osteoblasts die in the composition of new matrix[59] and the more their activity is stimulated, the more of them die.[60, 61] Since the number of times a bone cell can reproduce itself is fixed, the reproduction capacity will be exhausted sooner if too much calcium continues to be absorbed. This is because the supply of osteoblasts will become exhausted and both bone and bone matrix will begin to break down. The lack of pre-calcified bone matrix, as well as bone, will lead to the development of pores – and hence osteoporosis.

The problem arises only if too much calcium is actually absorbed into the bones, and, as we have discussed in Chapter 2, the absorption rate decreases when we consume more calcium than we need. There is some evidence, however, that if we continually consume too much calcium, the absorption rate cannot be decreased enough. For example, an American study has shown that a group of girls whose calcium intake was increased fivefold absorbed twice as much calcium as previously.[62] The purpose of absorbing extra, unwanted calcium into the bones would be to prevent blood-calcium levels from rising too much. The excess dietary calcium is temporarily stored in the bones, prior to excretion, in order to prevent damage to essential body processes, including heart function (as discussed in Chapter 2).

The problem of continually consuming too much calcium has been likened to building a house which keeps having far more bricks delivered to the builders than are needed.[63] Eventually, in order to be able to watch television or clean the house, the extra bricks must be thrown out. This involves the builders in excessive and unnecessary work, and eventually they become exhausted. Similarly, the osteoblasts – which have to carry the calcium into the bone, like the house-builders with their bricks – become exhausted and die prematurely.

There is experimental evidence from animal models that moderate calcium levels are healthier because where less calcium is consumed the bone cells age more slowly. A low calcium intake during adolescence has been shown to retard and prolong longitudinal bone growth in rats.[64] According to this school of thought, bone mineral density can be increased over the short term by consuming large quantities of calcium, although it is argued that over the longer term this will have the effect of exhausting the bones sooner. Hence, countries with the highest average bone mineral density also have the highest incidence of hip fracture.[65]

If bone mineral density is low because an individual has consumed relatively little calcium throughout their life, then any increased bone mineral density will be protective. Even where calcium intakes are very low, there may still be enough calcium for the calcification of bone matrix.[66] However, if the bone mineral density is low as a result of exhausted osteoblasts, and has been reduced as a result of the lack of new bone matrix, the bones will become osteoporotic.

Calcium supplements are another commonly promulgated remedy for osteoporosis, but this has been shown in clinical and epidemiological studies to be of very dubious value.[67]

AN INITIAL CLUE!

Other evidence that strongly suggests that osteoporosis is not a disease of calcium deficiency relates to the calcium content of human breast milk. Human beings need more calcium as babies than at any other stage of their lives, because babies' bones are weak and need to be calcified. Mother's milk is considered by most health professionals to be the best possible food for babies. It contains all the calcium (and other nutrients) babies need in their first two years, and babies fed on mother's milk increase their bone-mineral density to normal levels. Mother's milk, however, contains less calcium than hazel or brazil nuts, or figs, blackberries, oranges or kiwi fruit (Table 3.2, Figure 3.3).

TABLE 3.2 **CALCIUM IN FOODS, mg PER 100 g**[68]			
Food	**Ca**	**Food**	**Ca**
Cow's milk	*119*	*Human milk*	*32*
Hazelnuts	226	Coconut	20
Egg yolks	140	Grapes	18
Brazil nuts	132	Apricots	16
Olives, green	96	Pineapple	16
Walnuts	87	Plums	14
Figs	54	Salmon	13
Blackberries	44	Mackerel	12
Oranges	42	Mango	12
Raspberries	40	Watermelon	11
Kiwi fruit	38	Avocado	10
Mandarin	33	Banana	9

Despite the official recommendations for calcium intake (Chapter 1, Table 1.1) infants, and adults, including the elderly, need less calcium than babies (per kg bodyweight), so it would seem logical that their food does not need to contain as much calcium as mother's milk. But cow's milk contains a whopping three to four times as much calcium as mother's milk! Surely this amount exceeds human needs.

Many natural foods contain similar or higher levels of calcium to that found in mother's milk, so that we do not need to be obsessed with increasing our calcium intake, although, as we shall discuss later, there are other very beneficial changes that we can make to our diet to protect us against osteoporosis.

FIGURE 3.3 **CALCIUM CONTENTS OF DIFFERENT FOODS* IN mg PER 100 G, RELATIVE TO HUMAN BREAST MILK**

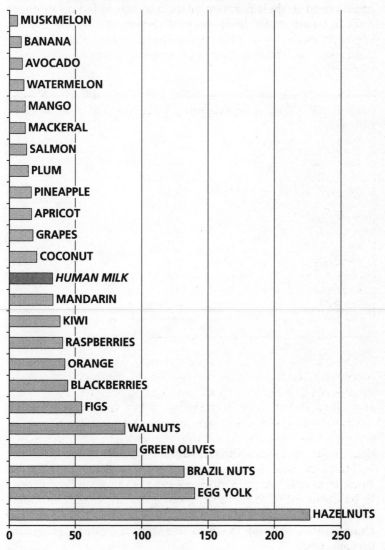

* http://www.4.waisays.com

ALCOHOL

Let us, next, use the dataset on hip fracture incidence (HFI) and information from the FAO sheets to look at the evidence on alcohol consumption as a potential cause of osteoporosis. In Figure 3.4 we have plotted alcohol consumption per person for the same 33 countries we have been examining. Interestingly

FIGURE 3.4 **RELATIONSHIP BETWEEN HIP FRACTURE INCIDENCE*
AND CONSUMPTION OF ALCOHOLIC BEVERAGES†, FOR 33
COUNTRIES**

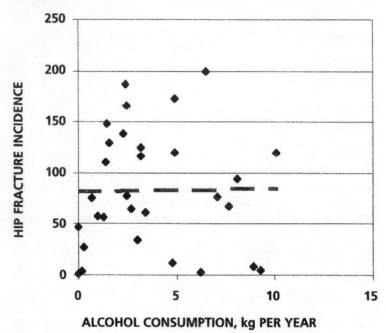

ALCOHOL CONSUMPTION, kg PER YEAR

* Frassetto, L.A., Todd, K.M., Morris, R.C. Jr and Sebastian, A. 2000. Worldwide incidence of hip fracture in elderly women: relation to consumption of animal and vegetable foods. *Journal of Gerontology: Medical Sciences*, 55A, 10, M585–M592.

† *Food Balance Sheets*, 1991. Statistics Division of the Economic and Social Policy Department. Food and Agriculture Organisation of the United Nations.

and surprisingly, the data suggest that there is no relationship whatsoever between HFI and average alcohol intake. This mismatch may be partly due to cultural factors, in that the HFI data are for women over fifty years of age, whereas the data on alcohol consumption represent the average for the whole population and in some cultures women do not consume alcohol. Nevertheless if alcohol were such an important factor in the development of osteoporosis, as suggested by conventional medical sources, one would expect some evidence of a relationship, rather than the total scatter apparent in Figure 3.4. Of course, where people drink an excessive quantity of alcohol, especially if they obtain most of their calories from this source so that they become deficient in a whole range of nutrients, it is very likely that they will increase their risk of osteoporosis. Nevertheless, the data once again suggest that one of the factors considered by conventional medicine to be of crucial importance in osteoporosis is not the key to the epidemic increasingly affecting post-menopausal women in Western countries.

VITAMIN D

One of the other conventional messages for the prevention and treatment of osteoporosis is to ensure adequate intake of vitamin D in order to promote calcium absorption. An important source of vitamin D for most people is sunlight. In sunlight, the body transforms cholesterol into vitamin D (a hormone called cholecalciferol), which is essential for the absorption of calcium (and phosphate) from the intestine into the blood. It also facilitates bone mineralisation. (Vitamin D deficiency in young children results in enlarged wrists and ankles and bowed legs, a condition known as rickets or osteomalacia.)

Osteoporosis incidence, however, shows no relationship with sunlight. Italy has a much higher average amount of sun than Poland, but hip-fracture incidence in Italy is much higher[69] than in Poland,[70] and in Italy 25 per cent more dairy products are consumed.[71] Kuwait is extremely sunny, but dairy consumption is high[72] and osteoporosis incidence there is similar to that of Great Britain and France.[73] In 52 per cent of Saudi Arabian females examined, vitamin D level was extremely low (because of clothes that block almost all sunlight), but their bones were not affected.[74]

According to some research, consumption of some fish and/or egg yolk once in a while provides all of the vitamin D needed – even in Greenland, Canada or Northern Europe.[75] As already indicated in Chapter 1, too much supplementary vitamin D can cause health problems. It can increase the blood-calcium level,[76, 77] and the extra calcium can precipitate in arteries, causing arteriosclerosis, and on the outside of the bones, causing bone deformities.[78, 79, 80, 81, 82, 83] Vitamin D is considered further in Chapter 6, Lifestyle Factor 1.

ON THE TRAIL

So, if the osteoporosis epidemic affecting elderly people in Western industrialised countries is not caused by calcium or vitamin D deficiency or alcohol consumption, what is it caused by? Let us return to the data on hip fracture incidence rate in 33 countries collected by Frassetto and her co-workers[84] and look at the relationships between HFI and the dietary factors that they investigated, again using the FAO datasheets. They first plotted HFI against total animal protein intake (Figure 3.5). This shows that the more animal protein there is in the diet the higher is the HFI. This relationship, shown in Table 3.3 and Figure 3.5, confirms the earlier findings of Abelow and others[85] that the incidence of hip fracture in women over the age of fifty is directly correlated with the consumption of animal protein. Frassetto and her colleagues also plotted HFI against total vegetable protein intake and found evidence that vegetable protein is protective. However, the most remarkable relationship that they found is that shown by their plot of HFI against the ratio of animal protein to vegetable protein in the diet (Figure 3.6).

The eleven countries with the lowest HFI also have the lowest animal protein consumption per person, with a vegetable-to-animal protein ratio greater than 1. In contrast, among the eleven countries in the highest group for HFI (more than 116 per 100,000 person years) animal protein intake exceeded vegetable protein intake in all of the countries except

FIGURE 3.5 **RELATIONSHIP BETWEEN HIP FRACTURE INCIDENCE (HFI) AND CONSUMPTION OF ANIMAL PROTEIN (AP), FOR 33 COUNTRIES***

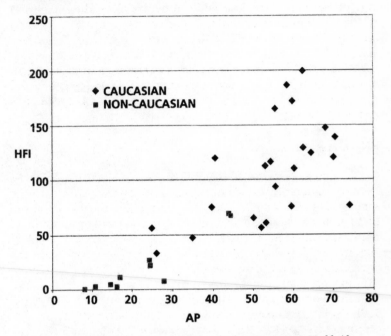

* Frassetto, L.A., Todd, K.M., Morris, R.C. Jr and Sebastian, A. 2000. Worldwide incidence of hip fracture in elderly women: relation to consumption of animal and vegetable foods. *Journal of Gerontology: Medical Sciences*, 55A, 10, M585–M592.

Portugal. Looking at the full set of 33 countries studied (Table 3.3), the data clearly show that the higher the total protein in the diet, the higher the total animal protein and the lower the total vegetable protein intake, the higher the HFI.

These plots by Frassetto and co-workers[86] show convincingly that globally HFI in women aged fifty and over is directly related to the ratio of animal to vegetable protein consumed. Hence they associate HFI with the acid–alkaline balance of the diet. They relate this to the direct effect of animal food consumption

FIGURE 3.6 **RELATIONSHIP BETWEEN HIP FRACTURE INCIDENCE (HFI) AND RATIO OF VEGETABLE TO ANIMAL PROTEIN (VP/AP) IN THE DIET, FOR 33 COUNTRIES***

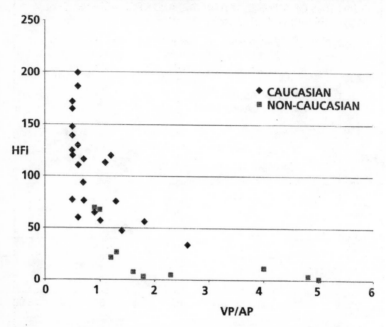

* Frassetto, L.A., Todd, K.M., Morris, R.C. Jr and Sebastian, A. 2000. Worldwide incidence of hip fracture in elderly women: relation to consumption of animal and vegetable foods. *Journal of Gerontology: Medical Sciences*, 55A, 10, M585–M592.

in increasing acid production in the body and the inverse effect of vegetable food consumption in increasing base production in the body. That is to say, the higher the proportion of animal protein in the diet relative to protein of vegetable origin, the greater the risk of hip fracture. In contrast, the more vegetable protein consumed, the lower the risk. It is worth noting that the results for countries with predominantly Causcasian populations (23 in total) were similar to those obtained in the primary analysis of all countries.

TABLE 3.3 **AGE-STANDARDISED RATES OF HIP FRACTURE INCIDENCE (HFI) IN 33 COUNTRIES**, COMPARED WITH THE QUANTITIES OF ANIMAL PROTEIN (AP) AND VEGETABLE PROTEIN (VP) IN THE DIET AND THE RATIO VP/AP*

Country	HFI per 100,000 person-years	Animal protein intake (AP) (g/day)	Vegetable protein intake (VP) (g/day)	VP/AP
Nigeria	0.8	8.1	40.2	5.0
China	2.9	10.7	51.2	4.8
New Guinea	3.1	16.3	29.7	1.8
Thailand	5.0	14.7	34.3	2.3
South Africa	7.7	27.8	45.4	1.6
Korea	11.5	16.9	68.6	4.0
Singapore	21.6	24.5	30.2	1.2
Malaysia	26.6	24.3	32.7	1.3
Yugoslavia	33.5	26.1	67.8	2.6
Saudi Arabia	47.3	35.0	49.1	1.4
Chile	56.8	25.0	44.8	1.8
Italy	57.2	52.1	51.9	1.0
Holland	60.7	53.3	33.6	0.6
Spain	65.1	50.1	44.1	0.9
Japan	67.3	44.3	42.5	1.0
Hong Kong	69.2	44.0	36.7	0.9
Israel	75.5	39.7	51.0	1.3
Ireland	76.0	59.6	41.7	0.7
France	77.0	74.2	36.7	0.5
Finland	93.5	55.7	36.4	0.7
Canada	110.3	60.4	34.7	0.6
Crete	113.0	53.1	55.9	1.1
United Kingdom	116.5	54.4	36.3	0.7
Portugal	119.8	40.7	48.9	1.2
United States	120.3	70.1	32.9	0.5
Australia	124.8	64.7	33.3	0.5
Switzerland	129.4	62.6	35.2	0.6
New Zealand	139.0	70.6	34.3	0.5
Argentina	147.8	68.2	36.9	0.5
Denmark	165.1	55.6	30.5	0.5
Sweden	172.0	59.9	29.8	0.5
Norway	186.7	58.6	34.0	0.6
Germany	199.3	62.4	35.3	0.6

The data are for women over the age of fifty. HFI is expressed as fractures per 100,000 person years, standardised to the age-group distribution of women in the USA in 1987.

* Frassetto, L.A., Todd, K.M., Morris, R.C. Jr and Sebastian, A. 2000. Worldwide incidence of hip fracture in elderly women: relation to consumption of animal and vegetable foods. *Journal of Gerontology: Medical Sciences*, 55A, 10, M585–M592.

Frassetto and her co-workers[87] suggest that the relatively high incidence of hip fractures in women in industrialised countries is caused, at least in part, by the cumulative effects on the bone of the body's chronic retention of too much of the high dietary net acid load. This high dietary net acid load, in turn, is the result of disproportionate consumption of animal (acid precursors) relative to vegetable (base precursors) foods. The degree of acid retention is determined partly by the size of the excess acid load caused by the diet. It is also partly attributed to the ability of the kidney, which declines with increasing age, to regulate the net acid–base balance of the body, resulting in increasing degrees of chronic low-grade metabolic acidosis in older people. Moderation of acid food consumption and an increased ratio of vegetable to animal food in the diet appear to confer a protective effect.

The association with animal protein has been known for a considerable time. Observations from epidemiological studies carried out in different countries as long ago as 1970 show that the higher the dietary intake of animal protein, the more common is osteoporosis.[88] Also, WHO statistics show that osteoporosis is most common in those countries where animal (including dairy) products are consumed in the largest quantities – the USA, Finland, Sweden and the United Kingdom.[89] Also, after reviewing studies on the link between protein intake and urinary calcium loss, R. P. Heaney found that as the consumption of protein increases, so does the amount of calcium lost in the urine.[90] He notes that this effect has been documented in several different studies and adds 'the net effect is such that if protein intake is doubled, without changing the intake of other nutrients, urinary calcium content increases by about 50 per cent.'[91] The new evidence of Frassetto and co-workers, however, suggests that it is the proportion of animal to vegetable protein in the diet that is the most important factor. The new work also indicates the bone-protective effects of consuming vegetables.

More recently Professor Sellmeyer and her co-workers,[92] also from the University of California, San Francisco, tested the idea that a high ratio of animal to vegetable protein in the diet increases bone loss and the risk of fracture. Their study, which complements the global studies of both Abelow and co-workers, and Frassetto and co-workers, was based on white American women. Interestingly Sellmeyer and her co-workers found no relationship between the dietary ratio of animal to vegetable protein and bone mineral density as measured by DEXA. However, women who had a high proportion of animal to vegetable protein in their diet had both a higher rate of bone loss at the 'neck' of the femur or thigh bone, where hip fractures generally occur, and a greater risk of suffering hip fracture. Other metabolic and lifestyle factors have been considered, by other authors, to affect the acidity of the body. For example, infection and smoking have been considered to make the body more acid.[93, 94] Conversely, exercise is thought, initially, to make the body more alkaline, but if continued beyond a comfortable level it can become acid forming, as lactic acid levels build up.[95, 96]

However, the associations between diet and bone loss and hip fracture risk, found by Sellmeyer and her co-workers, were unaffected by other potential risk factors including age, weight, oestrogen use, tobacco smoking status, alcohol use, exercise, total calcium intake or total protein intake. Yet again, some of the sacred cows of the osteoporosis gurus appear irrelevant when compared with the impact of the consumption of a typical Western diet. Certainly, it is not a lack of calcium that appears to be at the root of the problem. Indeed, as we shall see in the next chapter, eminent scientists now believe that it is the Western diet, high in supposedly health-promoting cereals, high in animal protein, including calcium-packed cheeses, and low in fruit and vegetables that is responsible for the 'epidemic' of osteoporosis. This diet is believed to produce so much acid in our bodies that, over time, it rots the bones and muscles. Anthony Sebastian, also of the University of California, San Francisco, was quoted in New Scientist[97] as saying of the acid generated in our bodies by such a diet: 'It's like water running over a rock: it's not going to look like it's even touching the rock, but over time it will erode it away.' A former director of the British Geological Survey, Sir Kingsley Dunham, once referred to the Pennine Hills that run north–south through northern

England as the backbone of England. Like the human backbone, the Pennine hills are largely made up of calcium minerals which form limestone. Rainwater is naturally slightly acid and has become increasingly so as a result of increasing industrialisation. Over time, the Pennines have been partly dissolved by the acid waters, leaving behind great cave and cavern systems.

A FINAL QUOTE

The association between the intake of animal protein and fracture rates appears to be as strong as the association between cigarette smoking and lung cancer.[98]

Dr T. Colin Campbell,
Professor Emeritus at Cornell University, New York State,
and a pioneer of dietary epidemiology.

KEY POINTS

● Data on Hip Fracture Incidence (HFI) – the most reliable indicator of osteoporosis – from 33 countries around the world shows that those living on a traditional Western diet have up to 200 times the HFI of countries such as Nigeria and China. The differences do not reflect genetic factors.
● Many data suggest that a high dairy/high calcium intake is associated with a higher incidence of osteoporosis.
● Many foods from oranges to nuts and eggs contain more calcium than human breast milk, so giving up dairy does not mean inadequate calcium intake.
● The main association between HFI and diet is the ratio of vegetable protein to animal protein. Where this is high, HFI rates are very low. Conversely, where this ratio is low, there is a higher rate of bone loss, especially at the part of the thigh bone where hip fractures generally occur.

4 Balancing for Your Bones

In this chapter we present more detailed evidence on how to maintain the acid/alkaline balance in our bodies, which is crucially important for the health of our bones and muscles, and for our health generally. An imbalanced diet is one that is too high in animal protein and processed foods, with too little fruit and vegetables. We include a detailed chart of the acidity and alkalinity generated in the body by the metabolism of different kinds of foods and drinks. This information, derived from the latest scientific research, will help you to plan your own diet, while ensuring that it is balanced in terms of acidity and alkalinity. We also include a table of the calcium and magnesium contents of the same foodstuffs. Finally, we discuss some of the trace minerals that are essential for bone health and recommend good dietary sources for them.

NUTRITION AND ACID–ALKALINE BALANCE

In December 2001, Douglas Fox published an article in *New Scientist* entitled 'Hard Cheese'.[1] He began by stating, 'All that Gouda and Cheddar you eat to keep your bones hard and strong may be having the opposite effect.' He went on to explain that a growing number of nutritional scientists believe that the thinning of bone (and muscle) with age is actually related to modern Western diets – diets that appear healthy but 'are in reality setting the stage for an old age of hunched backs, hip fractures and withered muscles'.

The idea that an acid-producing diet might rot bone and muscle originated in the 1920s.[2] Doctors noticed that patients with failing kidneys (you will remember from Chapter 2 the important role of kidneys in acid excretion) had unusually fragile skeletons, but when they were given bicarbonate to alleviate stomach-acid build-up (one of the principal symptoms of kidney failure) their bones gradually grew sturdier.

Much later, in 1968, two Harvard Medical School physicians published a little-noticed letter in *The Lancet* suggesting that healthy people eating diets that produced too much acid in their bodies could be putting their bones at risk. The idea stemmed from a basic understanding of how the body deals with acid, and a back-of-the-envelope calculation.

As discussed in Chapter 3, keeping the blood at a slightly alkaline pH is a top priority for the body. This is because if the blood were to become too acid or too alkaline we would become ill and the range of pH that can be tolerated is extremely small (Chapter 2, Table 2.2). If the pH is not corrected, excessive acidity or alkalinity can lead to death.

In order to stop molecules such as enzymes from malfunctioning, the body keeps the pH of arterial blood very close to 7.4 – just slightly alkaline. The kidneys excrete excess acid in the urine, but if the pH becomes too low (more acid) a more drastic response is needed. At this stage the body compensates by breaking down bones (and muscles) to release carbonates, phosphates and ammonia, in order to neutralise the excess acidity. As discussed in Chapter 2, bone is not simply a structure that stops the body collapsing; it is also the principal storage system for alkaline minerals and bases that can neutralise excess acid in the diet.

The two Harvard researchers calculated that diets which are acid enough to leach just a few tens of mg of bicarbonate – equivalent to a few dimples on a golf ball – from the skeleton each day would have leached 15 per cent of the skeleton's entire mineral mass after one decade.

According to Fox, this is a survival mechanism that is thought to have been acquired by early humans to deal with periods of excess acid caused by starvation and shortages of vegetables in harsh winters.[3] But while excess acid in the body was probably a short-lived problem for our hunter-gatherer ancestors – the minerals that were leached from their bones and muscles were quickly replenished – for many in the West today it is a chronic problem because of our continual consumption of highly acid-producing diets.

As discussed in Chapter 3, the amount and type of dietary protein ingested has been known for some time to affect bone-mineral loss after the menopause in women.[4] The first real evidence came from the Department of Home Economics, Andrews University, Berrien Springs, USA,[5] which reviewed several epidemiological studies relating to bone density and diet. The first survey involved 1,600 women in south-western Michigan and revealed that those who had followed a lacto-vegetarian diet for at least twenty years had lost only 18 per cent of their bone mineral by age eighty, whereas closely paired omnivores had lost 35 per cent (i.e. omnivores suffered almost double the bone loss of the vegetarian women).

A separate study of self-selected weighed food intake showed no statistical difference in the amount of calcium ingested. However there were distinct differences in the ratios of calcium to animal protein and the amount of acid generated by different foods in the diet.[6]

Even seemingly acid vegetables and fruits, such as lemons, actually produce large amounts of alkalis because they contain organic salts such as citrates, which are metabolised into bicarbonates. On the other hand, grain foods such as pasta and bread produce some acid because they are high in phosphorus, which the body turns into phosphoric acid. Other high-protein foods such as eggs, meat and cheese contain sulphur which is metabolised into sulphuric acid.

It is estimated that our consumption of acid-producing protein has increased by 50 per cent over the past forty years.[7] When we fail to compensate by eating enough fruit and vegetables (which contain bases to neutralise the acid) the body fluids become so acid that they leach alkalis from the skeleton and also attack the muscles to generate ammonia as a source of alkalis.

Calculations on the acid produced when food is metabolised confirm the epidemiological evidence.[8] According to Loren Cordain, an evolutionary biologist at Colorado State University (quoted in the *New Scientist* article[9]), our ancestors who were hunter-gatherers ate meat, but their carbohydrate was primarily from fruit and vegetables which countered the acid load. Today in industrialised countries the diet typically includes a lot of acid-producing meat, cheese and cereal-based products such as bread and pasta, with far too little fruit and vegetables to balance the acid generated by such high-protein diets.

Many vegetable foods which are high in protein, including soya and other beans and whole-grain cereals, also generate some acid, but in quantities that are easily balanced by eating some fruit and vegetables. These plant sources of protein also contain phyto-oestrogens which help to replace the body's own oestrogen after the menopause and are therefore protective of bone.

High-protein diets in general, and meat- and cheese-based diets in particular, lead, over time, to a gradual decrease in bone density. Even many vegetarians in industrialised countries consume too much protein, especially cheese (one of the most acid-forming foods) or yoghurt, and hence can also be affected by osteoporosis.[10]

According to Amrit Willis,[11] most Americans are eating an inverted diet of 80 per cent acid-forming foods and only 20 per cent alkali-forming foods. Willis quotes some of the findings in Dr Susan Lark's book, *The Chemistry of Success*. Dr Lark examined the statistics on the American diet produced by the Economic Research Service of the US Department of Agriculture (USDA). She added up the number of pounds of highly acid-forming foods that the average American eats per year and compared it with the average yearly intake of more alkali-forming foods. The ratio she discovered was an amazing 17:3 in favour of acid-forming foods. This highly acid-forming diet puts a great strain on the buffering systems of the body, especially the skeleton, to neutralise all the acid that is produced by such a diet.

In her book, Dr Lark states, 'As we age, our ability to maintain a slightly alkaline balance in our cells and tissues diminishes. All too many factors in modern life, including the standard American diet, also affect the acid–alkali balance in the body. Our diet is high in acidic and acid-creating foods, and the fast pace of life today increases acidity.'[12]

She goes on to say: 'Maintaining the cells and tissues of the body in their healthy, slightly alkaline state helps to prevent inflammation. In contrast, over-acidity promotes the onset of painful and disabling inflammatory conditions as diverse as colds, sinusitis, rheumatoid arthritis and interstitial cystitis.[13] A diet that is too acid can also lead to gallstones, kidney stones and gout.[14] As Baroody has stated starkly in his book *Alkalize or Die*, 'When this alkaline reserve is depleted, death follows.'[15]

We saw in Chapter 3 how research by eminent scientists in America has shown that the higher the proportion of animal protein in the diet relative to protein of vegetable origin, the greater the risk of hip fracture.[16, 17] These findings were attributed to the amount of acid produced in the body when the food is metabolised. As discussed above, foods of animal origin contain higher proportions of non-metallic elements such as sulphur and phosphorus, which create acids (sulphuric and phosphoric acids), while foods of vegetable origin are protective of bone because they contain alkaline elements such as calcium and bases such as bicarbonate, which help to alkalise the body. Most vegetables are rich in substances such as citrates and succinates (which the body metabolises to bicarbonate) – bases which mop up hydrogen ions. Vegetarian diets based on ingredients such as soya, lentils and other pulses and cereals as sources of protein yield significantly lower rates of acid production in the body than mixed meat and vegetable diets, even when the diets are equal in protein content. Diets that are predominantly of vegetable foods are frequently very well-balanced, yielding no net acid or alkaline residue in the body.[18] Renal net acid excretion (in urine) increases with increased intake of animal protein and decreases as vegetable protein increases.[19] Careful studies indicate that diet-dependent differences in acid production in the body are sufficiently large to disturb the acid–alkali equilibrium.[20, 21]

Evidently, people eating a typical Western diet are in a chronic state of acidosis,[22] and the kidneys do not dispose of the entire daily acid load, thereby imposing a chronic demand for base of skeletal origin.[23, 24] Because the degree of acidosis in the systemic circulation does not increase measurably from day to day,[25, 26, 27, 28] there must be an internal reservoir supplying base. Bone is the only base reservoir with sufficient capacity for such a mechanism to operate over a lifetime.[29] Over decades, the magnitude of daily positive acid balance may be sufficient to induce osteoporosis.[30, 31] Reducing the diet net acid load to nearly zero by supplementing the diet with alkaline/base improves calcium balance, reduces bone resorption, and stimulates bone formation.[32]

Before the Second World War, there was considerable interest in how the food we eat affects the acid–alkaline balance of the body. While the subject receives little attention in orthodox medical circles today, many alternative practitioners continue to place considerable stress on the acid–base balance characteristics of various diets. It is generally acknowledged that the food that is eaten is a major source of acid and alkali for the body.[33]

There has, nevertheless, been considerable confusion about which foods generate acid and which generate alkali. Initially, investigations into how different foods might affect the acid–alkaline balance involved burning various foods to ash in the laboratory and determining the pH of the resulting ash. These foods were then classified as acid, alkaline or neutral ash foods. An example is shown in Table 4.1.[34]

TABLE 4.1 **ACID, ALKALINE AND NEUTRAL ASH FOODS.**[36]
CHALLENGED: SEE TABLE 4.3 FOR CORRECT INFORMATION

Acid ash foods	Alkaline ash foods	Neutral ash foods
bread (grains)	cheese	arrowroot
cake	cream	butter
cereal	most fruit	candy
mayonnaise	jam	coffee
cranberries	milk	cornstarch
plums	almonds	lard
prunes	chestnuts	margarine
meat	coconut	vegetable oil
Brazil nuts	molasses	white sugar
walnuts	most vegetables	syrup
peanuts		tapioca
legumes		tea
corn		

In addition, famous naturopaths and alternative health practitioners such as Edgar Cayce and Bernard Jensen used acid- and alkaline-forming foods in their approach to disease, based on the reaction that they determined that foods would have in the body. These categories are shown in Table 4.2.[35]

These are just two of the many different charts available, and it is clear that there are considerable discrepancies. For example, in Table 4.1 butter is shown as being a neutral foodstuff while in Table 4.2 it is listed as an acid-forming food. Coffee is shown as a neutral-ash food in Table 4.1, but as acid-forming in Table 4.2. Note, however, that both charts show most dairy products as alkaline-ash or alkaline-forming foods. Some fruits such as plums, prunes, cranberries, rhubarb (not a fruit, but with a similar role in

---

TABLE 4.2 **ACID- AND ALKALINE-FORMING FOODS.**[37]
CHALLENGED: SEE TABLE 4.3 FOR CORRECT INFORMATION

Acid-forming foods	Alkaline-forming foods
All meat, poultry, eggs, and seafood	All fruits except those noted opposite
All foods made from cereal grains including breads, breakfast cereals, crackers, pasta and rice	All vegetables except beans, peas and lentils
Fat including salad oil, butter, margarine, lard etc.	Dairy products including milk, buttermilk, cheeses and yoghurt
Legumes including beans, peas, lentils and peanuts	
Fruits containing benzoic or oxalic acid including prunes, plums, cranberries, rhubarb and sour cherries	
Chocolate	
Coffee, tea and most soft drinks	
Sugar, syrup	
All true nuts	

the diet) and sour cherries were also said to be acid-forming since they contain either oxalic or benzoic acid, organic acids which are not completely broken down in the body.[38, 39, 40] So, if balancing our diet to leave little or no acid or alkaline residue is so important, where can we obtain reliable information?

A MODEL DIET

In 1995 a considerable amount of work on the acidity produced by foods after they have been metabolised was published by Thomas Remer and Friedrich Manz of the Institute of Child Nutrition at Dortmund in Germany.[41]

Because previous methods had failed to provide reliable estimates of the net acid loads produced by diets,[42] these scientists developed and tested a different, and totally new, method, based on computer calculation, for estimating the renal (kidney) net acid excretion (NAE) from nutrient intake data.[43] Scientists had known for several decades that the composition of the diet influenced the urine pH,[44] and clear experimental evidence had shown that it was possible to adjust the urine pH by changing the diet.[45, 46, 47]

The model that was developed by Remer and Manz takes into account the mineral and protein composition of foods, the average intestinal absorption rates of the different nutrients, sulphur metabolism, and urinary excretion of organic acids, and it proved to be able to predict the amount of acid excreted by the kidneys of experimental animals. In addition, the scientists used their findings to adjust the urine pH of healthy adults, using diet alone.[48] **For the first time, we have a truly scientific method for determining the acidity or alkalinity that foods generate in our bodies that can help us to balance our diets effectively.**

Since Remer and Manz were able to show a direct relationship between their calculations and dietary urine, they went on to calculate and specify the potential renal acid loads of many commonly consumed foods and to demonstrate how to use the data to predict the corresponding urine pH of people consuming particular diets. In addition to the dietetic prevention of osteoporosis, their results have important applications for the prevention of kidney stones and urinary-tract infections (see under 'Some other applications', page 77, below).

The results of the work, together with calculations for soya products, spices and herbs, kindly supplied by Dr Remer (personal communication to Jane Plant), are presented in Table 4.3.

The results obtained by Remer and Manz, using their computer model, are completely consistent with the findings of the epidemiological studies reviewed in Chapter 3 and earlier in this chapter. The results are expressed in units called PRALs (potential renal (kidney) acid loads) per 100 g portion of food, which are the end result of the metabolism of food in the body. The higher the PRAL value for the food, the more acid, and hence the more potentially damaging, it is predicted to be to bones and muscles unless balanced by adequate intakes of foods with negative PRAL values.

HARD CHEESE INDEED!

The PRAL values in Table 4.3 range from a maximum of 34.2 for parmesan cheese and a whopping 26.4 for other hard cheese, through 0 for fat and oils to a minimum of –62.4 for dried parsley. Among the raw (i.e. non-dried) fruits, the base-forming potential is similar to that of vegetables.

The lowest PRAL values are for certain herbs and spices, which are not normally eaten in large quantities, and for raisins. Apart from these, the lowest values are for fruits, fruit juices and vegetables (which are moderately to strongly alkaline) and alkali-rich, low-phosphorus beverages (i.e. beverages containing less than 30 mg per 100 g phosphorus and with sodium + potassium content several times higher than chloride content. The good news is that these beverages include both red and white wine.[49] These foods are followed by low-alkali beverages (including stout and draught beer, tea and soya milk), as well as fats and oils – all of which are essentially neutral). Moderately acid foods include most dairy products, as well as some types of bread and rice, and pulses such as peas and lentils. Acid and strongly acid foods include fish, meat and meat products, some cereals and soya products, eggs and, most importantly in view of the orthodox advice quoted in Chapter 1, cheeses. Some cheeses are very strongly acid, including cheddar-type reduced fat, processed cheese and parmesan cheese.

It is clear from Table 4.3 that the most potentially bone-damaging foods are therefore cheeses – especially hard cheeses. They are approximately three times more acid-generating than beef, for example. At the other end of the spectrum are many herbs and spices which have been used for a long time in Eastern cooking and which, if used in the correct quantities, help to neutralise the acid generated by meat, fish and cereals such as rice. The table makes it very clear why diets based on vegetable protein, which lack components with the extreme acidity of typical Western diets, are protective of bone and muscle. There are some surprises in the table. For example, most of the alcohol tested (which included wine and beer) appears not to be bone-damaging. This is consistent with the simple comparison we made in Chapter 3 of hip fracture incidence and alcohol intake, which suggested little, if any, relationship, and also the findings of Sellmeyer and her colleagues.[50]

On the other hand, dairy products are shown not to be alkaline-producing. For example, milk is shown not to have the moderately negative PRAL value suggested by previous work;[51] instead, it is moderately acid-generating. Hence, dairy products are not helpful in balancing the body pH. Indeed, all that calcium-packed cheese generates such large amounts of acid, according to the new data, that calcium and other alkaline bone minerals would be carried out of the body on the acid tide generated by a cheese sandwich unless it is accompanied by massive quantities of spinach and/or other large quantities of fruit or vegetables. According to Dr Remer (quoted in New Scientist[52]), this is because of the way cheese is made. Milk contains roughly equal proportions of acid- and base-producing nutrients, but to make cheese – especially hard cheese – the liquid that contains the base-forming constituents (the whey) is removed.

On the other hand, whole wheat – with a PRAL of + 1.8 – is shown to be much less acid-producing than previously thought.

The most acid-producing, and therefore most bone-damaging, foods consumed include hard and processed cheeses, egg yolk (so be careful with the egg mayonnaise!) and, to a less extent, canned and processed meats. The most protective foods because of their alkaline production in the body are fruit, vegetables, herbs and spices.

It is essential, however, to have some acid-forming foods in the diet or other conditions, caused by excessive alkalinity, can be induced: do not become so extreme in cutting out acid-forming foods that you become protein deficient. Also remember that every human being is unique. We do not all metabolise food in exactly the same way. Depending on our ancestry and our genes, we may have different nutritional requirements. Hence there are no hard and fast rules and we recommend you to use Table 4.3 as a guide to find a dietary regime which is suitable for you.

The new data are superior to the old acid-ash diet calculation methods[53, 54] and those based on current food tables,[55] which were unable to predict the urine pH levels produced by particular diets. Remer and Manz, in contrast, were able to demonstrate the validity of their method by accurately predicting urine pH levels in healthy men.[56] They also assert that their method will predict the pH of the urine of healthy women because there is no gender difference in renal acid excretion.[57, 58] Clearly the data provided by Remer and Manz are vitally important to mineral balance and skeletal metabolism in post-menopausal women.[59] It is worth mentioning some of the other applications of the information.

SOME OTHER APPLICATIONS

Interestingly, Remer and Manz suggest that diets can be changed to control the development of kidney stones, especially where these are confirmed as calcium phosphate or magnesium ammonium phosphate (struvite) stones. In these two cases, a generally accepted basic principle of treating the condition or preventing recurrence consists of urine acidification.

TABLE 4.3 POTENTIAL RENAL ACID LOAD (PRAL) OF FOODS AND BEVERAGES (RELATED TO 100 g PORTIONS)*

	Very strongly alkaline	Strongly alkaline	Alkaline	Moderately alkaline	Nearly neutral	Moderately acid	Acid	Strongly acid	Very strongly acid
	−20		−10	−5	−0.5	0.5	5	10	20
Herbs and spices	Parsley, dried −62.4 Basil, dried −57.9 Ginger −23	Curry powder −19.9 Black pepper −19.7		Chives −3.6					
Fruits and juices	Raisins −21		Blackcurrants −6.5 Bananas −5.5	Apricots −4.8 Kiwi fruit −4.1 Tomato Juice −3.8 Cherries −3.6 Orange juice −2.9 Pears −2.9 Pineapple −2.7 Oranges −2.7 Lemon juice −2.5 Peaches −2.4 Apple juice −2.2 Apples −2.2 Strawberries −2.2 Watermelon −1.9					
Vegetables		Spinach −14	Celery −5.2	Carrots, young −4.9 Zucchini −4.6 Cauliflower −4.0 Potatoes, old −4.0 Radish, red −3.7 Eggplant −3.4 Tomatoes −3.1 Beans, green −3.1 Lettuce −2.5 Chicory −2.0 Leeks −1.8 Lettuce, iceberg −1.6 Onions −1.5 Mushrooms −1.4 Peppers −1.4 Broccoli −1.2 Cucumber −0.8	Asparagus −0.4				
Beverages				Red wine −2.4 Mineral water (example) −1.8 Coffee −1.4 White wine, dry −1.2 Grape juice −1	Cocoa −0.4 Tea −0.3 Beer, draught −0.2 Beer, stout −0.1 Mineral water (example) −0.1 Cola 0.4	Beer, pale 0.9			

Food category						
Fats and oils			Margarine −0.5 Olive oil 0.0 Sunflower-seed oil 0.0			
Sugars, sweets and preserves		Marmalade −1.5	Honey −0.3 Sugar, white −0.3	Chocolate, milk 2.4 Madeira cake 3.7		
Legumes and nuts	Soya flour −5.9	Soya beans −4.7 Natto −3.2 Hazelnuts −2.8	Soya milk −0.3 Soya bean, sprouted raw 0.3	Peas 1.2 Mori-Nu tofu 2.0 Tofu 3.4 Lentils 3.5 Soya sauce 4.5	Miso 6.9 Tempeh 8.2 Tofu, prepared with calcium sulphate 8.3 Walnuts 6.8 Peanuts, plain 8.3		
Grain products				Rice, white, boiled 1.7 Bread, wheat wholemeal 1.8 Crispbread, rye 3.3 Bread, wheat, white 3.7 Bread, wheat, mixed 3.8 Bread, rye, mixed 4.0 Bread, rye 4.1 Rice, white 4.6	Rye flour, whole 5.9 Cornflakes 6.0 Noodles, egg 6.4 Spaghetti, white 6.5 Wheat Flour, white 6.9 Spaghetti, wholemeal 7.3 Wheat flour, Wholemeal 8.2	Oat flakes 10.7 Rice, brown 12.5	
Meat					Frankfurters 6.7 Beef, lean 7.8 Pork, lean 7.9 Chicken, meat 8.7 Steak, lean and fat 8.8 Veal 9.0 Turkey, meat 9.9	Luncheon meat 10.2 Liver sausage 10.6 Salami 11.6 Corned beef 13.2	
Fish and eggs				Eggwhites 1.1	Haddock, 6.8 Herring 7.0 Cod 7.1 Eggs, whole 8.2	Trout 10.8	Eggyolks 23.4
Dairy products				Butter 0.6 Ice cream 0.6 Milk, whole 0.7 Milk, evaporated 1.1 Creams, fresh, sour 1.2 Yoghurt, fruit 1.2 Yoghurt, plain 1.5 Soft cheese 4.3	Cottage cheese 8.7	Fresh cheese 11.1 Camembert 14.6 Cheese, Gouda 18.6 Hard cheese 19.2	Cheese, cheddar-type, reduced fat 26.4 Processed cheese 28.7 Parmesan 34.2

PRAL values are expressed in milli-equivalents of X per 100 g portion of food consumed, where X is the percentage of principal acids (chloride (Cl) + phosphate (PO_4) + sulphate (SO_4)) minus the percentage of principal bases (sodium (Na) + potassium (K) + calcium (Ca) + magnesium (Mg)) present in the food.

* Remer, T. and Manz, F. 1995. Potential renal acid load of foods and its influence on urine pH. *J Am Diet Assoc.*, 95, 791–797, and Remer, personal communication.

For struvite or calcium phosphate stones, both of which are poorly soluble at higher (alkaline) urine pH values, solubility can be increased, and precipitation inhibited by adequate decreases of urine pH. However, for patients with uric acid stones, adjusting urine pH to near 6.8 is recommended. Such changes in urine pH level can be achieved in healthy subjects, it is suggested, by purely dietary measures.[60, 61]

In a case of non-infectious calcium oxalate stones, a pH increase is considered helpful.[62, 63] Therefore, the recommended high fluid intake[64] should be achieved by drinking alkalising (i.e. potassium/alkali-rich, phosphorus poor) beverages such as tea, wine or beer. Do not drink coffee, because it contains relatively high amounts of oxalate, and excess intake seems to increase renal calcium losses.[65]

Some individuals digest and metabolise foods differently. This may determine whether a food leaves an acid or alkaline residue in the body. For example, certain foods containing organic acids, such as citrus fruits and tomatoes, which normally leave no acid residues, may be incompletely metabolised in some people and are thus acid-forming for these individuals. This may occur where stomach acid is low or thyroid activity is subnormal.[66] It is also worth noting that the PRAL data were generated using a library of the calculated contents of foods. There may be differences between the tabulated nutrient data (used for PRAL calculation) and the actual values of food and drink consumed due to inherent nutrient variations of natural foods and differences in their processing and preparation.[67]

Although the net acid balance of the diet is crucial to bone health, and probably to health generally, some trace nutrients are also essential to bone health. Some of these are considered in more detail below.

CALCIUM, MAGNESIUM AND ESSENTIAL TRACE ELEMENTS

The diet described in this book should be full of healthy vitamins and give rise to conditions in the digestive tract where vitamins such as B12 and K can be formed by gut flora. Vitamin D is a special case, considered in Chapter 3 and again in Chapter 6, Lifestyle Factor 1.

The calcium and magnesium contents of the foodstuffs listed in Table 4.3 are given in Table 4.4. It is clear that herbs and spices such as parsley and black pepper are good sources of both calcium and magnesium. Tofu, figs, nuts, wholemeal bread, green vegetables and some fish are also good sources. Eggs are a good source of calcium, and oat flakes of magnesium.

Trace elements cannot be guaranteed in foodstuffs, particularly in modern industrialised agriculture which depends on the use of inorganic fertilisers such as rock phosphate rather than fish meal or animal waste (as used by organic farmers). Moreover, some rock-phosphate fertilisers contain high levels of bone-damaging cadmium and uranium – and radioactive products of uranium – all of which tend to accumulate in bone. Here we shall describe the essential trace elements and some of the factors that control their levels in the body, using information mostly obtained from the World Health Organisation's book *Trace Elements in Human Nutrition and Health*,[68] unless otherwise stated. It is also worth remembering that the green revolution was based on nitrogen, potassium and phosphorus for plant growth, with no concern for the trace element content of crops.

Note that these are trace nutrients and that excess, as well as deficiency, can cause serious health problems.

IODINE
The major role of iodine in nutrition arises from the important part played by the thyroid hormones (of which it is an essential constituent) in the growth and development of humans and animals. Iodine-deficiency disorders (IDDs) occur particularly during periods of rapid growth and development (in foetuses, the newborn and children, and during puberty). IDDs include goitre (underactive thyroid hormone production), which is usually associated with a large swelling in the front of the neck, and inadequate brain development in the unborn child (cretinism). Iodine is also now strongly implicated in the development of Kashin-Beck (or Big Bone) disease.

TABLE 4.4 **CALCIUM AND MAGNESIUM CONTENTS OF SELECTED FOODSTUFFS***

Food	Calcium mg per 100 g	Magnesium mg per 100 g	Food	Calcium mg per 100 g	Magnesium mg per 100 g
Herbs and spices			Lime juice	8	5
Chilli, whole	18	24	Orange juice	10	10
Chilli, powder	269	154	Carrot juice	24	14
Cinnamon, ground	1217	43	Lemon juice	6	6
			Tomato juice	9	11
Curry, powder	500	250	Vegetable juice	11	11
Garlic, fresh	167	33			
Garlic, powder	71	71	*Vegetables*		
Oregano, ground	1600	267	Artichokes	45	60
Parsley, dried	1462	231	Asparagus	20	10
Pepper, black	429	190	Beans, baked	50	32
			Broccoli	48	25
Fruits			Chinese cabbage (bok choy)	93	11
Apples, with skin	7	5			
Apricots, dried	54	31	Cabbage, raw	47	16
Bananas	6	29	Cauliflower	22	15
Blackberries	32	20	Celery	40	11
Blueberries	6	5	Chickpeas	49	48
Dates	32	35	Cucumber	14	11
Figs	145	58	Eggplant	6	13
Grapefruit	12	9	Leeks	30	14
Grapes	11	6	Lettuce	36	5
Kiwi fruit	26	30	Mushrooms	6	10
Lemons, without peel	26	9	Onions	20	10
			Peppers	9	10
Oranges	40	10	Potatoes, baked, with skin	15	28
Paw paw (papaya)	24	10			
Peaches	5	7	Pumpkin	15	9
Pears	11	6	Radishes	22	0
Pineapple	7	14	Spinach	100	80
Plums	5	8	Tomatoes	5	11
Raspberries	22	18			
Raisins	49	33	*Beverages*		
Watermelon	8	11	Beer	5	6
			Cola, fizzy drink	4	1
Fruit juices			Coffee	3	4
Apple juice, no additives	7	3	Expresso coffee	2	80
			Ginger ale	3	1
Grape juice, no additives	9	10	Lime/lemon, fizzy drink	2	1
Grapefruit juice, no sugar	7	10	Teas, various	2	1
			Water, club soda	5	1

Food	Calcium mg per 100 g	Magnesium mg per 100 g	Food	Calcium mg per 100 g	Magnesium mg per 100 g
Wine, dessert	8	9	Spaghetti, wholemeal	15	30
Wine, red	8	13			
Wine, white	9	10			
			Meat		
Fats and oils			Beef, sirloin steak	11	32
Margarine	28	0	Beef, ground	31	20
Olive oil	0	0	Chicken, meat only	13	22
Sunflower seed oil	0	0	Corned beef	12	14
			Frankfurters	13	13
Sugars, sweets and preserves			Pork, luncheon meat	7	20
Chocolate, milk	191	59	Pork, leg	14	22
Honey	5	0	Salami	10	15
Cake	70	10	Turkey	5	22
Jams, preserves, marmalade	20	5	Veal, rib	11	22
			Fish and eggs		
Legumes and nuts			Cod, Atlantic	21	41
Beans, green	49	24	Eggs, whole, large	48	10
Hazelnuts	113	162	Eggs, whites	6	12
Miso	65	42	Eggs, yolks	139	6
Peanuts, salted	53	226	Haddock	42	51
Soya, beans	102	86	Herring	76	8
Soya, milk	4	19	Trout	86	32
Soya, sauce	19	31			
Tempeh	65	42	*Dairy products*		
Tofu	162	46	Butter	21	0
			Cheese, camembert	387	21
Grain products					
Bread, rye	72	41	Cheese, cheddar	721	28
Bread, white	108	24	Cheese, low fat	186	13
Bread, wholemeal	80	96	Cheese, parmesan	1380	60
Cornflakes	7	11			
Crispbread – crackers	117	25	Cheese, processed	617	28
Flour, rye	72	41	Cheese, cottage	60	5
Flour, white	108	24	Cream	67	7
Flour, wholemeal	80	96	Ice cream	127	14
Noodles	12	19	Milk, low fat	123	14
Oat flakes	59	235	Milk, whole	119	13
Rice, brown	10	43	Milk, evaporated	290	11
Rice, white	19	12	Yoghurt, fruit	152	15
Spaghetti, white	7	18	Yoghurt, plain	183	17

* US Dept of Agriculture – Nutrient Database; Release 15.
http://www.nal.usda.gov/fnic/foodcomp

Kashin-Beck disease is a debilitating condition which affects several million people in central Asia and central Africa, where the usual diet often lacks two essential trace elements, iodine and selenium. In Asia it occurs in a crescent-shaped region extending from south-east Siberia to south-west China. The principal pathological change associated with the disease is the degradation and death of cartilage. The pain and restricted movement caused by the disease make it difficult for sufferers to work and the disease has serious social and economic consequences, especially as it affects the poor. Recent studies[69] have emphasised the importance of iodine deficiency as the major risk factor in the disease. They suggest that iodine deficiency impairs thyroid activity, which in turn slows bone growth and causes joints to stiffen. Iodine has not normally been considered an essential element for bone health, but the interconnections between different hormone systems are increasingly being recognised as important. Selenium-iodine interaction in the thyroid and inter-relationships between iodine, selenium and vitamin E also affect how the immune system controls and reacts to certain viruses and other pathogens such as bacteria and fungi. Prevention of the disease in China now involves supplying iodine and selenium, ensuring adequate quantities of vitamins, and improved storage of food (since a microorganism has also been implicated in the development of the disease).

The main sources of iodine in the diet are marine foods such as marine fish, shellfish and seaweed. Vegetables can contain significant amounts of iodine when grown on soils rich in organic matter, especially where they are fertilised with fish waste or are near to the sea (where rainwater contains iodine). It is for this reason that IDDs and Kashin-Beck disease tend to occur in the centre of large continents such as Africa and Asia where there is little marine influence. Cooking can greatly reduce the level of iodine in food, because it tends to escape with the steam. The usual recommended level of iodine in the diet is 100 to 150 mcg per day, although if the diet contains large quantities of cassava, maize (corn), bamboo, sweet potatoes, lima beans, millet or cabbage, all of which can affect thyroid function, higher levels – 200 to 300 mcg – are recommended. Taking high levels of inorganic iodine as pills or in fortified bread, salt or milk is not recommended because, as with all trace elements, high levels can be toxic. Some Japanese people eat so much fish and seaweed that their daily intake of iodine is extremely high (50,000 to 80,000 mcg per day) and some of them develop symptoms of toxicity also.

ZINC

Zinc is essential for all forms of life. It is the second most important trace element, after iron, in the human diet. The principal features of zinc deficiency are growth retardation, delayed sexual maturation, dermatitis around the mouth and anus, alopecia, appetite failure and behavioural changes. For our purpose, of developing healthy bones, zinc deficiency causes delay in skeletal maturation. It enhances the action of vitamin D and is required for the synthesis of protein in bone tissue as well as the formation of osteoblasts and osteoclasts – the cells responsible for bone remodelling.[70] Zinc is present in all tissues and fluids of the body. The total body content is estimated to be only about 2 g. About 30 per cent of this is stored in the skeleton, which is probably the way the body maintains control of levels of this vitally important nutrient in tissue and blood. As we have seen in Chapter 2, calcium and magnesium are, similarly, stored in the skeleton, though many other nutrients are stored in the liver.

Lean red meat is one of the best sources of zinc, and its zinc is present in a highly bioavailable form. In general, the darker the meat the higher the zinc levels – so chicken legs have higher zinc contents than breast meat. Whole grains and legumes are also good sources of total zinc. Energy sources such as fats, oils, sugar and alcohol contain very little zinc. Green leafy vegetables and fruits are only modest sources of zinc, because of their high water content.

Taking an inorganic supplement containing as little as 50 mg of zinc per day can induce problems with copper metabolism and, in some people, copper deficiency. It is better to obtain zinc from the diet, when the body has a better chance of maintaining appropriate levels.

It has been suggested that a diet which is high in cereals and pulses containing a fibre called phytate can have an adverse effect on absorption of zinc and other trace elements. Normal intake of unrefined cereals and pulses does not cause a problem,[71] but it is recommended that people do not add additional fibre such as bran to any of their meals. Fermenting grains to make substances such as tempeh (from fermented soya beans) soya sauce, miso (from fermented soya or cereals such as barley) or beer overcomes the problem.

SELENIUM

Until recently, the only known role for selenium in mammals was that it acted together with vitamin E as an antioxidant. (Think how butter becomes rancid if it becomes oxidised; selenium and vitamin E help to prevent this happening in the human body.) There is, however, growing evidence of the involvement of selenium in the synthesis of thyroid hormones, as discussed above. Selenium deficiency has also been linked to heart disease and, more importantly for our purpose, to Kashin-Beck disease. Selenium and vitamin E deficiency are also implicated in liver and muscle degeneration in animals. Once again, it must be emphasised that selenium is toxic at high levels, with the development of problems with the skin and the nervous system. Selenium poisoning in humans is characterised primarily by hair loss and changes in the shape of finger and toe nails. It has been suggested that selenium protects against cancer, but the available evidence on this is inconclusive. Unrefined cereals, soya, yeast, meat and garlic can be good sources of selenium.

COPPER

Copper enzymes (catalysts) are involved in many processes in the body. Copper has a key role in the development of the skeleton, as well as the heart, the circulatory system and the nervous system including the brain. One of the most important aspects of copper physiology is its role in activating the enzyme which cross-links collagen and elastin in connective tissue. As we have seen, collagen makes up much of the soft framework of the skeleton, while elastin is important in the soft discs between the spinal vertebrae.[72] Of particular importance in considering bone health is the role of copper in enzymes which are involved in the formation of essential components of the body, especially the connective tissues of bone (and blood vessels). A variety of symptoms have been reported in animals with copper deficiency, and many of these symptoms also occur in humans. They include a type of anaemia, loss of pigmentation of the hair and skin, problems with blood vessels and the metabolism of cholesterol and, of great importance here, skeletal fragility and osteoporosis, even in infants. Indeed the WHO book[73] shows two photographs of X-rays of infants a few months old with clearly developed osteopenia caused by copper deficiency. Microscopic evidence of bone disease has been reported in mildly copper-deficient animals. Some of the early classical experiments into copper deficiency were carried out by feeding animals milk diets.[74] However, copper poisoning can also occur.

Copper is widely distributed in plants and animals. Good dietary sources of copper (more than 2 mcg per g) include seafood, liver and kidney (but use these only from organically reared animals), legumes (such as peas and beans) and nuts. Refined cereals and sugar are low in this essential element, as is dairy produce. There is evidence that many factors can cause problems with copper uptake during digestion. These include taking high levels of vitamin C (more than 1500 mg per day),[75, 76] high levels of calcium and phosphorus (more than 2 g per day),[77, 78] high levels of cadmium, high intakes of inorganic iron or lead, very high sugar levels, high levels of inorganic zinc, and diets high in sulphur and the trace element molybdenum. Many Western diets are low in copper, and milk and dairy products are poor sources, while lactose may interfere with copper metabolism. This may be one of the reasons why current recommendations for a diet high in dairy produce to prevent osteoporosis may actually be detrimental to health.[79]

CHROMIUM

Chromium-deficient animals exhibit glucose intolerance similar to diabetes mellitus, high levels of cholesterol and triglycerides in the blood, increased incidence of plaques on major blood vessels, problems with the cornea of the eye, decreased fertility and sperm count and, of importance for our purposes, impaired growth. Chromium levels in the diet are more likely to be low where high quantities of refined food are consumed, because considerable quantities are lost in food processing. Some meats, whole-grain products, pulses, spices (especially black pepper) and brewer's yeast are the best sources of chromium, while dairy products, fruit and vegetables contain very little.

MANGANESE

Manganese deficiency in animals can cause impaired growth, reproductive problems and skeletal abnormalities. Manganese stimulates the production of the soft framework of the skeleton (osteoid) on which calcification takes place.[80] It has been suggested that the high incidence of cartilage disorders in children in parts of southern Africa may reflect low intakes of manganese.[81] Good dietary sources include unrefined cereals, nuts, leafy vegetables and tea. Diets high in refined carbohydrates, meat and dairy products are low in manganese. Indian diets high in foods of unrefined plant origin supply an average of 8.3 mg of manganese per day, whereas diets high in refined foods in America provide less than 1.75 mg per day.[82]

SILICON

Silicon is also vitally important for the normal development of connective tissue and bone, with poorly formed joints and reduced contents of cartilage and collagen in deficient animals. Silicon has a role in the early stages of bone mineralisation and is thought to be located in osteoblasts. The silicon content of animal tissues declines with age. The best sources of silicon are foods of plant origin, with some of the highest levels in cereals.

BORON

Boron in the diet helps the metabolism of the steroid hormones, oestrogen and testosterone, in humans and animals.[83] It is necessary for vitamin D synthesis and is highly concentrated in bone. Foods of plant origin, especially fruit, leafy vegetables, nuts, legumes, wine, cider and beer are high in boron. Meat, fish and dairy products are poor sources. It has been noted that where consumption of plant foods is high, boron levels may be high and this may be one of the reasons why a vegetable-rich diet is preventative of osteoporosis.

PHOSPHORUS

Phosphorus is the second most abundant mineral in bone. The calcium:phosphorus ratio should be 2.5:1. Excess phosphorus can cause osteoporosis.[84] It decreases calcium absorption and generates acid in the body, leading to bone loss.

It is common in the diet and deficiencies are highly unlikely. The Western diet in general is particularly high in phosphorus, especially when many commercial fizzy drinks are consumed.

MAGNESIUM

Magnesium is the third most abundant mineral in bone. It also assists calcium absorption and bone mineralisation. It is abundant in nuts, seeds, grains and vegetables of all sorts. In green plants, magnesium is to chlorophyll what iron is to haemoglobin in blood. Food processing removes much of the magnesium from food. Meat and dairy products are low in magnesium, with poor magnesium/calcium ratios. Sugar and alcohol increase excretion of magnesium and can lead to deficiency. According to J. R. Lee,[85] chocolate is high in magnesium and chocolate craving can be a sign of deficiency. Table 4.4 gives the magnesium contents of common foodstuffs.

VITAMINS

Some vitamins are particularly important for bone health and these are plentiful in the Plant Programme. Particular bone problems[86] concerning vitamins include the following: vitamin K is essential in the mineralisation of bone and overuse of antibiotics can kill off the organisms in the intestines which produce it; folic acid (one of the B family of vitamins) decreases levels of a damaging protein called homocysteine, implicated in causing osteoporosis; alcohol interferes with absorption of folic acid, and contraceptive pills can cause deficiency of this vitamin; vitamin D is a special case and is considered further in Chapter 6, Lifestyle Factor 1.

SOME GOOD FOOD SOURCES OF ESSENTIAL TRACE ELEMENTS

Trace element	Good food source
Chromium	Black pepper, brewer's yeast, mushrooms, prunes, raisins, nuts, asparagus
Copper	Liver, kidneys, shellfish, whole-grain cereals, legumes, nuts and chocolate (but choose dairy-free dark chocolate)
Magnesium	Nuts, legumes, green vegetables (chlorophyll), cereals, chocolate, hard water, beer
Manganese	Cereals, nuts, ginger, tea. Very low in animal foods
Selenium	Wheat, soya, yeast, meat, garlic
Zinc	Related to protein components in animal and vegetable foods. Follows colour of meat (higher in darker meat)
Boron	Fruits and berries
Iodine	All sea food

KEY POINTS

● Eminent scientists have shown that it is the Western diet high in animal protein, including cheese, and cereals, and low in vegetables and fruit that produces so much acid it leaches our bones, leaving them fragile and damaged and at increased risk of fracture (osteoporosis).

● New scientifically based studies clearly show the most acid-generating and hence bone-damaging foods are cheeses (especially hard cheeses) and, to a lesser extent, meat, eggs, fish and cereals.

● Such studies show the most alkaline-generating bone-protective foods include spices such as ginger and garlic, herbs, vegetables, dried and fresh fruit (including citrus fruit and tomatoes!). Some minerals, such as calcium, magnesium, copper and selenium, and vitamins such as Vitamin K, folic acid and Vitamin D are also essential for bone health – but it is best to obtain these from a healthy diet rather than by popping pills.

● In this and other chapters we advise you to keep to 60 per cent alkaline-forming and 40 per cent acid-forming foods to prevent osteoporosis, and 80 per cent alkaline-forming and 20 per cent acid-forming foods for treatment.

● Studies of the American diet indicate a typical ratio of 80–85 per cent acid-forming and 15–20 per cent alkaline-forming foods.

5 The 'Osteoporosis Plant Programme' – The Food Factors

In this chapter we describe the basis of the diet that we recommend to prevent and treat osteoporosis. The diet is based on that of China and has evolved over thousands of years. We give seven Food Factors which are important for bone health and describe how to make the changes to your diet. The Osteoporosis Plant Programme is very similar to the Plant Programme as described in our previous books, but with increased emphasis on balancing acid- and alkali-generating foods.

BACKGROUND TO THE DIET – *THE CHINESE WAY*

The 'Osteoporosis Plant Programme' diet, like the previous 'Plant Programme',[1, 2] is based on a modified Chinese, or East Asian diet. Like Chinese medicine, this diet is based on thousands of years of observation and practical experience. It has been handed down from one generation to the next, making use of the pictogram system of writing, which was developed early in their history. Chinese writing has evolved progressively into the sophisticated system in use today (an educated person in China today is expected to know at least 10,000 different pictograms) and, like the diet that is recommended here, continues to evolve.

Legend in China describes how Emperor Shen Nung, known as 'the divine farmer' and revered as the founder of Chinese agriculture, set out in 3494 BC to discover the healing properties of plants. Each day he would taste various plants to determine their properties – poisoning himself several times in the process, so that he also had to find many antidotes. This story of Emperor Shen Nung may well be a metaphor for the trial and error method of the discovery of the properties of plants, but there is little doubt that Chinese agriculture and medicine are derived from knowledge accumulated over the last three to five thousand years. It is worth recalling that China had reached a considerable level of sophistication while the people of the British Isles were still emerging from the Stone Age. There are several philosophies central to Chinese thinking, which have survived all religious, social and political influences, including communism. The philosophy of yin–yang, representing opposite but complementary forces throughout the universe, dates back to somewhere between 1000 and 700 BC. Later, the philosophy of Confucius (551 to 479 BC) focussed on an orderly relationship between society and natural cycles. In the West we are only just starting to come to grips with the idea that protection of the natural world could be in our own interests and those of generations to come (the concept of 'sustainable development', following the 1989 Brundtland report[3]).

We do not intend to develop here the full concept of yin and yang, but it is relevant to explore something of the philosophy. For example, yin is associated with the moon, form and rest, while yang is associated with the sun, energy and activity. Yin is feminine, introvert and vegetable. Yang is male, extrovert and animal. Every food has a yin or yang aspect, and Chinese living and medicine are based on balancing yin and yang.

Yang foods are generally stimulating and energy-giving (warm), and include such foods as sugar, ginger and cayenne pepper. Yin foods are cooling and include many fruits. Extremes of yin and yang are believed to produce opposite effects. Seaweed, for example, is considered a yin food – but it is salty. On the other hand, salt, when used as a seasoning, is considered to bring out the yang quality of food.

To those used to modern Western diets and medicine, all this probably sounds like mumbo-jumbo, but in reality, it is a memorable way of capturing well-documented concepts! Let us give an example based on our own subject of the Earth sciences to illustrate why we strongly believe that observation, which is the basis on which Chinese agriculture, eating and medicine has developed, is sound.

In Japan, people used to believe that their islands were situated on the back of a large turtle. When the turtle became angry, it shook itself, causing massive shock waves, which destroyed buildings and communications. We now know that there is no angry turtle, but that the Japanese Islands occur in a particularly unstable geological setting. The so-called 'ring of fire' that encircles the Pacific Ocean is marked by volcanoes and earthquakes caused by deep geological forces. Despite the explanation of the angry turtle being seen now as just a quaint superstition, it was a metaphor which allowed the Japanese to develop an excellent and practical response to the earthquakes that frequently shattered their towns and villages. They lived in small houses of one or two stories, built of light wood with thin rice paper walls and paper lampshades, and they slept in roll-up beds called futons that were easy to carry around. This minimalist lifestyle was far better protection to human life than the highly engineered structures developed today, even when we know so very much more about the Earth and earthquakes and earthquake engineering. Just think of the terrible loss of life and destruction of property caused by the 1995 Kobe earthquake.

The Chinese diet and Chinese medicine should be viewed in a similar light. The basis may sound strange to modern scientists, but the observations provide excellent responses to nutritional and environmental problems and have sustained the Chinese population for thousands of years. The Chinese even separated their waste streams so that only animal or human waste was recycled back into agricultural land, minimising contamination and the need for fertiliser. The Chinese diet, which has recently been studied in great depth by a team of eminent scientists from Cornell, Oxford and Beijing universities, has been shown to be one of the healthiest diets in the world. Contrast this diet evolved over thousands of years with the very many 'healthy' diets that are promulgated on the basis of single-issue science, such as the body's response to insulin, or the need for a few isolated nutrients (vitamin C or calcium, for example).

Of course, it is not just Asian traditions that have messages for today's generation. Let us take four examples of how folklore and customs have grown up and become part of a culture that works to protect people from environmental problems in Britain. In some parts of Scotland there are granites which are naturally radioactive, and consequently emit small amounts of the radioactive gas radon. Radon is colourless and odourless, but if people are exposed to it for long periods of time, then the incidence of a type of lung cancer increases. When Jane worked in north-east Scotland in the 1970s she noticed that Scottish people, especially from Aberdeenshire (her husband is from Aberdeenshire) are always keen to be in very well-ventilated rooms, ideally sleeping with the windows open, even on the coldest of nights. Good ventilation is, of course, the best defence against dangerous accumulations of radon gas.

Another example relates to the origins of the rim of pastry around the Cornish pastry. This is said to have been a response by the local community to observations that miners working in the tin mines developed 'stomach palsy' (which was probably stomach cancer). In addition to tin, the tin mines in Cornwall contain arsenic and uranium minerals, both potentially cancer-forming. When the miners ate their food with dirty hands they would ingest small particles of these potentially damaging chemicals. A practical response developed over the years – the Cornish pasty acquired a rim of pastry which forms a 'handle' that was traditionally discarded by the miners.

Also while working in Scotland early in her career, Jane noticed that many locals would run the water for a long time before filling the kettle – especially in the morning. Again, this is a custom, which has grown up that forms a very good defence against dissolved lead. This can result from the naturally acidic water in parts of Scotland leaching lead from the plumbing systems in old houses.

We recall that our grandmothers' generation used bicarbonate of soda a great deal in cooking, especially in boiling vegetables. Our own generation has made fun of this, but maybe there was a good reason for it. A pilot study into the link between an acid diet and osteoporosis carried out by Dr Anthony Sebastian used potassium bicarbonate (like baking soda) to neutralise the acid produced by diet.[4] According to

Sebastian, 'The effects were major.' The women treated with the bicarbonate lost 27 per cent less calcium in their urine than controls and all chemical indicators suggested it was because less bone was being broken down. The daily dose of bicarbonate also reduced muscle breakdown. Other similar evidence comes from experience of patients undergoing dialysis.

In each case, most people would probably be unable to give a scientific explanation for their traditional customs and behaviour. When questioned about the water, for example, they would say that 'it would have turned stale overnight'. Despite not understanding the real scientific basis of environmental problems that caused ill health, these communities nevertheless developed protective behaviour that was passed down through the generations. It is this kind of well-tried, observation-based depth of tradition, particularly from China and other parts of Asia, that forms the principles of the Osteoporosis Plant Programme diet described here.

PRINCIPLES OF THE DIET

We previously explained the scientific principles of a healthy diet, based on that of China, in *Your Life in Your Hands* and *The Plant Programme*. We are not going to go into the details of the scientific basis of the diet here, but it is worth looking in a little more detail at the Eastern diet in order to understand the principles of this chapter.

The diet is based on the traditional diet of China for the following reasons:

● Chinese people, living on their traditional diet, have one of the lowest recorded rates of hip fracture incidence in the world.
● Their diet has evolved over a long period of time and has been thoroughly documented and referenced. The diet is not a new fad based on the latest biological or chemical theory, but has evolved over more than 5000 years as a sustainable system of nutrition and agriculture by one of the most biologically successful people on Earth.

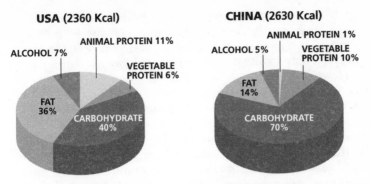

COMPARISON OF US AND EASTERN DIETS*

* From T. Colin Campbell and Chen Junshi's papers on Diet and Chronic Degenerative Disease, published in 1994.

● It has a very high vegetable protein to animal protein ratio. The Chinese diet has a ratio of vegetable protein to animal protein of 10:1. This compares to a ratio of 1:2 or worse in the USA and Germany, which are among the countries with the highest recorded incidence of hip fracture.

Typically, people in China do not eat dairy produce and the composition of their diet is very different from a typical Western diet in several other respects, for example:

● The Chinese take in more calories than do Americans[5] (but are much less obese).
● Only 14 per cent of calories in the average Chinese diet is from fat, compared to almost 36 per cent in the West.
● Animal protein makes up 11 per cent of the diet of the average American but only 1 per cent of the average Chinese (and a high proportion of that is from fish, eggs, chicken, duck or pork, rather than beef).
● The intake of alcohol in the Chinese diet is 5 per cent of total calories, which is similar to that of the USA, where it makes up approximately 7 per cent of total calories.

● Vegetables such as soya are the main source of protein in China giving a fibre intake of 34 g a day on average with no evidence of iron or other mineral deficiency, while in the USA the average fibre intake is only 10 to 12 g a day.

There are many scare stories about soya being circulated, mostly as unsubstantiated assertions on the Internet. We can find no convincing evidence that it causes adverse health effects. Indeed, authorities such as the Royal Society conclude that the phytoestrogens contained in soya are protective against cancer. Phytoestrogens are common in many foods, including all other peas and beans (close relatives of the soya bean), berries, whole grains and nuts. The Chinese diet is based heavily on soya and (at the risk of being repetitive) their rates of osteoporosis and bone fracture are among the lowest in the world.

Furthermore, in Japan a healthy diet is believed to be based on eating at least thirty different ingredients a day. Compare this with the diet of the average American, for whom 40 per cent of all that they consume is from dairy.

There are several reasons why the traditional Chinese diet is likely to prevent osteoporosis. First is that it contains no dairy. Milk has calcium levels that are excessive for humans as well as high levels of growth factors such as IGF-1 and EPO, which act as osteogenic proteins and may promote excessive bone remodelling. Milk also concentrates hormone-mimicking pollutants from the environment which could directly or indirectly damage bone.

The Chinese diet is also:
● high in phyto-oestrogens which are protective of bone
● low in fat
● high in natural fibre

THE FOOD FACTORS

The Osteoporosis Plant Programme is therefore based on the following seven Food Factors:

FOOD FACTOR 1 TO ACHIEVE A PROPER BALANCE
BETWEEN FOOD THAT IS ACID-GENERATING AND FOOD
THAT IS ALKALINE/BASE-GENERATING

HOW?
● Use Table 4.3 to balance animal foods (meat, fish and eggs)
and some pulses and cereals high in protein, with other
vegetable foods (including fruit, vegetables, herbs and spices).
● Completely eliminate all cheese, which is made from the
acid-forming component of milk and can generate three times
more acid, weight for weight, than beef.
● Avoid commercial fizzy drinks, many of which contain
excessive levels of phosphorus.

FOOD FACTOR 2 TO REDUCE THE INTAKE OF HORMONES
AND GROWTH FACTORS FROM FOOD THAT COULD CAUSE
OVERACTIVE BONE REMODELLING, ESPECIALLY AFTER
THE MENOPAUSE

HOW?
● Eliminate all dairy produce, including the meat of dairy
animals.
● Cut down on the amount of meat eaten – it should comprise
less than 10 per cent of daily intake for prevention and
treatment of osteoporosis.
● Ensure that meat is cooked slowly and thoroughly. Meat that
is raw inside contains hormones and growth factors, which
would otherwise be broken down during cooking (while
burning meat on the outside forms cancer-forming chemicals).
● Replace animal protein, especially dairy, with soya-based
food, and cereals and pulses. Meals that combine cereals and
pulses such as beans on toast or the Jamaican dish, rice and
peas, provide the full range of proteins needed by the human
body – but remember to eat some alkali-forming foods as well.

FOOD FACTOR 3 TO REDUCE THE INTAKE OF MAN-MADE
CHEMICALS FOR WHICH THERE IS EVIDENCE FOR, OR A
SUSPICION OF, ENDOCRINE-DISRUPTING ACTIVITY

These are suspected of causing problems with the thyroid, sex and other glands and could directly or indirectly affect bone. Hormone-disrupting chemicals are persistent and bioaccumulate, becoming particularly concentrated in certain foods such as dairy fat and fish-liver oils (the latter are good sources of vitamin D). See Chapter 6, Lifestyle Factor 1.

HOW?

● Avoid all dairy produce, certain fish-liver oils and farmed fish, especially carnivorous fish such as salmon (newly published research[6] shows that farmed salmon contains high levels of PCBs (polychlorinated biphenyls) and detectable levels of contaminants such as brominated flame retardants and the pesticides DDT and hexachlorocyclohexane).

● Eat only organically produced food, especially in the case of fat meats such as pork and duck, and discard the fat and skin before or after cooking. Food grown to the standards of the Soil Association is likely to have lower levels of cadmium (page 124) because sewage sludge cannot be used and the amount of cadmium in rock phosphate is prescribed. If you are in the USA, limit the amount of meat you eat, because anabolic steroids are still used there in livestock farming. In the UK they were perhaps an important route of human exposure in the 1950s to 1970s via residues in meat.

● Do not use plastic, especially soft plastic wrappings, or eat food from cans with plastic linings. Minimise your intake of food from cans generally.

● Filter tap water through charcoal, then boil it and store it in glass bottles.

● Drink liquids stored in glass with cork or aluminium seals, but not in plastic bottles.

FOOD FACTOR 4 INCREASE THE PROPORTION OF FOOD THAT IS PROTECTIVE OF BONE

HOW?

● Eat as much fresh organic vegetables and fruit as possible and from as wide a range as possible. Eat red vegetables such as tomatoes, red peppers and chillies; cruciferous vegetables such as bok choy, cauliflower and broccoli; and orange vegetables, including peppers, carrots and pumpkin.

● Eat lots of fresh herbs and spices also to alkalise the body.

● Eat vegetables as fresh and raw as possible and have at least five large portions of fruit and vegetables as salads or juices every day. The UK Government recommendation of five portions a day, which includes prepared fruit and vegetables, is completely inadequate for healthy living – one portion should be at least one piece of fresh fruit or a cup of raw vegetables. The aim should be to keep to a ratio of vegetables plus fruit to protein of about 60:40 for prevention and 80:20 if you have active osteoporosis.

● Eat a diet rich in phyto-estrogens, including soya and other beans and peas, whole-grain cereals including flax, nuts and berries such as cranberries, and sprouting seeds, especially alfalfa and beansprouts.

● Eat spices, especially with meat, fish and egg dishes since they help to counteract the acidity of such foods.

● Eat lots of garlic, onions and chives which are alkaline and have many other health benefits.

● Drink lots of green tea – the Chinese do.

FOOD FACTOR 5 ENSURE THAT YOU CONSUME ADEQUATE QUANTITIES OF THE KEY NUTRIENTS IN A BIO-AVAILABLE FORM, SO THAT A SIGNIFICANT PROPORTION CAN BE ABSORBED BY THE BODY

This is especially true of nutrients such as calcium, magnesium, boron, copper, iodine, manganese, selenium and zinc, all of which have important roles for the health of the skeleton, some for the crystalline minerals and some for the soft matrix (osteoid).

HOW?

● Eat more fresh or lightly cooked vegetables, fruit (including berries), nuts, seeds, seaweed, fish and shellfish.

● Have some brewer's yeast and Icelandic kelp every day (follow the instructions on the packet or bottle and ensure you take the correct dose).

● Take a good quality selenium supplement but be careful not to overdose.
● Follow the Japanese rule of eating at least thirty different ingredients a day.

FOOD FACTOR 6 ELIMINATE OR REDUCE TO A MINIMUM FOOD THAT HAS BEEN REFINED, PRESERVED OR OVERCOOKED, OR CONTAINS CHEMICAL ADDITIVES
In such foods, the content of fibre, vitamins, minerals, natural colours or other natural constituents have been removed or reduced. Be especially vigilant in avoiding man-made chemical substances, including artificial vitamins or minerals.

HOW?
● Cut out or cut down on manufactured convenience food especially anything with E-numbers in it. Frozen foods are usually OK and there is an increasing range of organically produced food available in bottles, jars and cans, which are fine occasionally.
● Use molasses, unrefined sugar, rice or maple syrup, or honey, rather than refined sugar (this includes all white sugars, and some refined sugars that have had brown colouring added).
● Use brown unrefined flour and pasta.
● Ensure that everything is as fresh, natural and unaltered as possible.
● Use as little salt as possible; if you must use it only have a little sea salt.
● Substitute herbal teas such as camomile, fennel, peppermint, clover and green tea for black tea and coffee (which is high in caffeine). A study of women aged 36 to 45 found that those who drank two cups of coffee a day suffered a net calcium loss of 22 mg per day. Reducing this to one cup daily reduced the loss to just 6 mg daily.[7]
● Do not drink too much alcohol, though the occasional beer or quality (preferably organic vegan) wine is fine.
● Eat good freshly made food to avoid the need for vitamin or mineral supplements.

● Never have food or drinks that contain man-made sweeteners such as saccharine or aspartame. Many diet drinks and food additives contain these substances.

FOOD FACTOR 7 PROVIDE MAXIMUM CHOICE AND VARIETY SO THAT HEALTHY EATING CAN BE MAINTAINED WITHOUT TOO MUCH RELIANCE ON ANY ONE FOOD SUBSTANCE

HOW?
● Have at least thirty different ingredients a day.
● Use herbs and spices to add flavour and balance acids generated by food, stress or modern living.

All this might sound a bit daunting, but when you have adjusted and are preparing and eating the great meals described in Section 2 of this book, we believe you will be a convert for life – especially when your health and appearance begin to improve. Anyway, we have done all the hard work of selection for you. All you need to do is to follow the shopping and cooking principles for the delicious meals described in Section 2 to help prevent or treat osteoporosis.

6 Lifestyle Factors

There are several other things, apart from diet, that you can change to help cut your risk of developing osteoporosis. Here we explain why you should make the changes, which range from taking appropriate exercise to avoiding bone-damaging chemicals, and how to make the changes successfully. We also include simple ideas to reduce the risk of fractures if you already suffer from osteoporosis.

LIFESTYLE FACTOR 1
VITAMIN AND MINERAL SUPPLEMENTS

It is preferable to eat whole foods, because problems can arise when we try to separate food into constituent parts or to change the structure of the natural molecules that produce beneficial effects. In some foods, like carrots, garlic and ginger, it is the whole package of natural chemicals that works together to benefit our health far more effectively than eating man-made copies of one particular constituent. We believe that eating good food is a far safer way of ensuring adequate vitamin and mineral intake than taking man-made pills (often synthesised from coal or petroleum derivatives). It is also important to remember that taking too much of one or other man-made supplement can cause a deficiency elsewhere in the diet. Let us use copper as an example since, as you will remember from Chapter 4, it is an essential element for the health of the soft (collagen) matrix of bone. There is evidence that high intakes (more than 1500 mg per day) of ascorbic acid (vitamin C) may restrict copper absorption[1, 2] and that intakes of calcium and/or phosphorus of more than 2 g per day increase faecal losses of copper.[3, 4] Also the bioavailability of copper has been found to decrease at levels of zinc supplementation (of more than 100 mg zinc per day).[5]

The supplements we are most encouraged to take to ward off osteoporosis are vitamin D and calcium.

VITAMIN D

A deficiency of vitamin D can occur when dietary intake is inadequate, when there is limited exposure to sunlight, when the kidney cannot convert vitamin D to its active form, or when it cannot be absorbed adequately from the gastrointestinal tract.

Vitamin D deficiency,[6] which occurs more often in post-menopausal women and older people in America,[7, 8, 9, 10, 11] has been associated with greater incidence of hip fractures.[12] A greater vitamin D intake has been associated with less bone loss in older women.[13] Since bone loss increases the risk of fractures, vitamin D supplementation may help prevent fractures resulting from osteoporosis.

In one group of women with hip fractures, 50 per cent were found to have signs of vitamin D deficiency. Treatment of deficiency[14] can decrease the incidence of hip fracture. It has been suggested that daily supplementation with 20 mcg of vitamin D may reduce the risk of osteoporotic fractures in elderly people with low blood levels of the vitamin.[15] The best natural food sources are oily fish and fish oils. Vegans usually obtain dietary vitamin D from fortified foods including soya milk, margarine and some breakfast cereals.

Exposure to sunlight is an important source of vitamin D, which is synthesised in the skin, depending on season, latitude, time of day, cloud cover, smog and the use of sunscreen designed to cut ultraviolet exposure.

There is a high health risk associated with consuming too much vitamin D.[16] Vitamin D toxicity can cause nausea, vomiting, poor appetite, constipation, weakness and weight loss.[17] It can also raise levels of blood calcium causing mental confusion and heart rhythm abnormalities. Vitamin D toxicity can also cause calcium and phosphate deposition in soft tissues, including the kidney. Consuming too much vitamin D is unlikely unless large amounts of fish liver oils are consumed. It is more likely to occur from taking too much of the vitamin in supplements.[18] We prefer to use fish oils, as necessary, but a recent survey[19] showed that several leading brands contained levels of PCBs and dioxins that could lead consumers to exceed safe levels of intake. One of the UK's market leaders (Seven

Seas) has the lowest levels due to its absorption-based purification process.

You should discuss your need for vitamin D supplementation with your physician, as part of an overall plan to prevent and/or treat osteoporosis.

CALCIUM

We certainly do not take calcium tablets. Indeed, we have both tried taking them and they gave both of us unpleasant and closely similar symptoms of nausea, heartburn and other gastrointestinal problems.

This is what happened to Jane. During the early stages of writing this book, she began to be brainwashed by the calcium propaganda and thought that since she had had no dairy produce for nine years she should try taking calcium tablets. She bought high-quality calcium and magnesium tablets, followed the instructions on the container and took them with food before her main meal in the evening. After a day or so, she began to feel quite sick with symptoms including heartburn shortly after her evening meal. Initially it did not occur to her that it could be the heavily marketed calcium and magnesium pill that was causing her problem. Eventually the smell of the pill was so strong to her that she started retching before putting it in her mouth. Finally the penny dropped and she gave up the calcium tablet, and within a couple of days all was well. But this started her thinking.

What occurred to Jane was this. Here is my stomach, full of acid, trying to digest my food, and what have I done – thrown in a large dollop of alkaline elements (calcium and magnesium) which will effectively neutralise the acid. So, what did my stomach have to do? It had to turn out even more acid, which probably reached parts of the digestive tract not appropriately lined to resist acids. The stomach is meant to be a bag of acid (see Chapter 2). That is why it works, to kill bacteria and to enable us to absorb acid-soluble components in food.

What about all those advertisements, particularly in America, trying to persuade us that if our stomachs are full of acid we should take antacids? It is now known that stomach ulcers can be caused by infections such as the bacterium *Helicobacter pylori*. In this situation the stomach overproduces acid to try to kill the bugs off. If you have acid indigestion or stomach ulcers, discuss it with your physician, who can arrange for a test for a possible infection and treat you with antibiotics if it is positive. If the tests are negative, and your doctor prescribes antacids you may need to remind them (yes, really!) that for the stomach to function properly it should be a bag of very strong acid. Trying to reduce or neutralise the acid may actually be the cause of the problem.

Back to bones, however. We believe our bodies were telling us, loud and clear, not to take extra calcium because we were getting adequate amounts from our diet. If Jane could have been persuaded to take such stuff by propaganda and once again have been saved further distress by her scientific know-how, we cannot help wondering how many other people are suffering side effects from taking calcium-magnesium pills or, indeed, other strong antacids that they do not need and which may well be making matters worse. See also the section on aluminium (page 127).

What we both learned was that if you follow the Plant Programme diet your own body will tell you that you do not need to take extra calcium-magnesium pills. Instead, look at the contents of calcium and magnesium in the foodstuffs listed in Table 4.4 (and the other vitamin and mineral sources you need to consume to maintain healthy bones: see Chapter 4) and ensure that you are taking enough of them by adjusting your diet as necessary.

FOOD SUPPLEMENTS WE USE OR WOULD USE

● Brewer's yeast (follow the manufacturer's instructions for dosage)
● Icelandic kelp (follow the manufacturer's instructions for dosage)
● Royal jelly from organic beekeepers
● Cod liver oil (in winter), purified to remove PCBs and dioxins
● Selenium supplement (occasionally)
● Balanced omega 3-6-9 oils
● Red clover, from herbalists

LIFESTYLE FACTOR 2 WEIGHT, SHAPE AND APPEARANCE

One well-known observation is that obesity gives protection against osteoporosis. This is thought to be because obese people have high levels of a hormone called leptin[20, 21, 22, 23, 24, 25, 26] which inhibits bone turnover by inhibiting osteoblast activity.[27, 28, 29, 30]

Obesity, however, causes very many other serious disease problems and is not recommended.

On the other hand, efforts to become unduly thin at any age are unhealthy and potentially bone-damaging. We saw in Chapter 1 how eating disorders are an important risk factor for osteoporosis. Many of us at the present time would like to be tall, thin, willowy blondes because that is the type of beauty that is now in fashion, just as in Rubens's time the fashion was for large fleshy females. Once again we must try to resist the conscious and subconscious brainwashing by advertising and the media as to what our body shape should be – brainwashing which drives people of all ages to try to slim excessively. We should try to accept our basic shape and work to achieve optimum weight and shape with a sensible diet and exercise plan. The Osteoporosis Plant Programme and the recipes included here are sensible and should help you to become the weight that is right for you. With appropriate exercise this can help you also to be the shape you were meant to be. Particularly after the menopause, slimming regimes that are too extreme can leave people looking unattractive, gaunt and ill, and where excessive protein is consumed as a means of losing weight both bones and muscles can be damaged. Eat healthily by following the Osteoporosis Plant Programme regime.

Many of the letters we receive about individual responses to the Plant Programme mention how much better people look and feel after just a few weeks or months of following this regime.

LIFESTYLE FACTOR 3 MEDICATION

We discussed in Chapter 1 how people with long-term illness – associated with the thyroid or pituitary gland, for example – can develop osteoporosis if the disease is untreated. On the other hand, many drug treatments, if used over a long period of time, can damage bone and are considered a risk factor for osteoporosis. Some medications are essential, and you should discuss with your doctor the relative risks of treatment and non-treatment. We suggest that, instead of simply suppressing the symptoms of, say, acne, eczema, psoriasis or asthma, you try the Plant Programme diet. If that does not work, try excluding wheat and other gluten sources. You could also ask to be referred to a specialist in food allergies and intolerances to find out the triggers of your condition. Gill's teenage years were made miserable by acne – which started when she introduced cheese into her diet and went away when she stopped eating it.

It seems ironic indeed that glucocorticoids are used to treat allergic symptoms which may be due to dairy consumption. When these are used over the long term, the risk of osteoporosis is known to increase (see Chapter 1, page 10) – and what is part of the advice to ward off osteoporosis? Have more dairy products! If you have any of the allergic or skin symptoms described, work with your doctor or qualified health professional using an exclusion diet (six weeks eliminating all dairy produce on the Plant Programme and if that does not work try next to eliminate gluten in the diet, gradually working through the big eight – see below, page 111) to pin down the fundamental cause of your allergy, noting that in a very small proportion of sufferers soya can be the culprit. When you have identified the underlying problem – and there is a very high probability that it will be dairy produce or gluten – keep to that regime and, with the agreement – and only with the full agreement – of your health professional, stop taking the pills and potions.

According to the website of the US Food and Drug Administration (FDA),[31] a food allergy, or hypersensitivity, is an abnormal response to a food triggered by the immune system. Many people often have gas, bloating or other unpleasant reactions to something they eat, but this is not a true allergic response. Such a reaction is called 'food intolerance'. Lactose (milk sugar) intolerance is very common, especially among non-Caucasians. This is of particular concern since it is used as the matrix or filler for many orthodox and herbal tablets. The FDA continues:

In food allergies, two parts of the immune response are involved, according to researchers at the National Institute of Allergy and Infectious Diseases. One is the production of an antibody called immunoglobulin E (IgE) that circulates in the blood. The other part is a type of cell called a mast cell. Mast cells occur in all body tissues but especially in areas that are typical sites of allergic reactions, including the nose, throat, lungs, skin, and gastrointestinal tract.

People usually inherit the ability to form IgE against food. Those more likely to develop food allergies come from families in which allergies such as hay fever, asthma or eczema are common.

A predisposed person must first be exposed to a specific food before IgE is formed. As this food is digested for the first time, tiny protein fragments prompt certain cells to produce specific IgE against that food. The IgE then attaches to the surface of mast cells. The next time the particular food is eaten, the protein interacts with the specific IgE on the mast cells and triggers the release of chemicals such as histamine that produce the symptoms of an allergic reaction.

If the mast cells release chemicals in the nose and throat, the allergic person may experience an itching tongue or mouth and may have trouble breathing or swallowing. If mast cells in the gastrointestinal tract are involved, the person may have diarrhoea or abdominal pain. Skin mast cells can produce hives or intense itching.

The food protein fragments responsible for an allergic reaction are not broken down by cooking or by stomach acids or enzymes that digest food. These proteins can cross the gastrointestinal lining, travel through the bloodstream and cause allergic reactions throughout the body.

The timing and location of an allergic reaction to food is affected by digestion. For example, an allergic person may first experience a severe itching of the tongue or 'tingling lips'. Vomiting, cramps or diarrhoea may follow. Later, as allergens enter the bloodstream and travel throughout the body, they can cause a drop in blood pressure or eczema, or asthma when they reach the lungs. The onset of these symptoms may vary from a few minutes to an hour or two after the food is eaten.

Over 170 foods have been documented in the scientific literature as causing allergic reactions.[32] Most sufferers are affected by the so-called 'big eight': milk, eggs, soya, wheat, peanuts, shellfish, fruits and tree nuts, which between them account for the great majority of food allergies.[33]

Pending legislation on allergens in manufactured foods, the UK Institute of Food Science & Technology makes the following recommendations for label warnings (to take the example of dairy): 'where calcium caseinate is the MSA (major serious allergen) concerned, the warning should read **"Contains MILK PROTEIN"**. It would be helpful to the purchaser to add to this category of warning the words **"to which some people may be allergic"**'.[34]

Many years ago, Jane was diagnosed by her doctor as having a condition called multiple chemical sensitivity. She appeared to be sensitive to almost everything, developing horrid rashes that made her look as if she had been through beds of nettles. The doctor tried to persuade her to use hydrocortisone cream to suppress the symptoms. She refused, and went to a private consultant allergist, who determined that she was sensitive to just two chemicals, formaldehyde and EDTA. These chemicals are used as preservatives in many products ranging from shampoos and cosmetics to furniture and clothing. Fortunately, with the help of her allergist and her own knowledge, she learned to avoid problems – for example by finding out the contents of cosmetics before buying them and by washing and thoroughly rinsing new clothes before wearing them (clothes are often treated with preservative to prevent the development of moulds and other growths). Nevertheless, a few years ago, after living on her dairy-free diet, she realised that all her sensitivities had gone.

Let us quote from a recent article in the *Sunday Times*[35] on the role of milk in allergies.

Hippocrates, the father of medicine, swore by milk-exclusion diets for curing all sorts: enfeebled babies, diarrhoea, skin complaints, wheezing, painful joints . . . As Hippocrates suspected, the white stuff [milk] is the commonest cause of childhood allergies. Standard medical advice is that such allergies usually desist by the age of three. But in a recent Finnish study, two thirds of a group of 56 infants diagnosed with cow's-milk allergy were still allergic and highly symptomatic at the age of 10. Other studies show that many children are milk allergic but don't know it. Reactions include runny noses, wheezing, coughing, ear infections, rashes and stomach upsets. When milk is withdrawn from their diet, symptoms improve or clear altogether, and reintroducing it leads to relapse in the majority. The chief culprits appear to be lactose and bovine protein.

LIFESTYLE FACTOR 4 ALCOHOL

According to research carried out by Dr Helen McDonald at the osteoporosis research unit at Aberdeen, who, with her team, looked at the lifestyles of 907 women over a seven-year period, moderate alcohol drinking could protect some women from developing osteoporosis.[36] The moderate levels of alcohol were equivalent to seven units a week: that is the equivalent of one glass of wine, half a pint of beer or one measure of spirits a day. Excessive alcohol consumption is unhealthy in many respects. As regards bone, Lee[37] states that, 'Whether from moderate alcohol toxicity to bone, magnesium loss, or other nutritional deficiency, osteoporosis is rampant among alcoholics.' We suggest that, ideally, moderate amounts of alcohol should be combined with food and enjoyed as part of a well-balanced social life as it is in southern Europe.

LIFESTYLE FACTOR 5 HELPING COUNTERACT OESTROGEN LOSS AT MENOPAUSE

As discussed in Chapter 1, most orthodox doctors in Western industrialised countries believe that the decline in oestrogen production at the menopause is one of the major factors in promoting osteoporosis in women over the age of fifty. So the simplistic solution was naturally to replace the oestrogen with oestrogen replacement therapy (ORT, or ERT in North America where oestrogen is spelled estrogen). It soon became clear, however, that this was associated with increased risk of endometrial cancer, which was attributed to giving unopposed oestrogen. This treatment was therefore replaced by tablets containing both oestrogen and progestins (hormone replacement therapy: HRT). Recent trials of one of these products has been abandoned, however, because the preliminary results, in line with the results of earlier studies, showed that the treatment under trial carried an increased risk for breast cancer, coronary heart disease and strokes (with an increased risk of 26 per cent, 23 per cent and 38 per cent respectively).[38]

Is there any alternative to HRT for the prevention or treatment of menopausal osteoporosis? Well, first of all let us remind ourselves that women in countries such as Nigeria and China have very low rates of osteoporosis. The word 'oestrogen' (from 'oestrus' meaning 'heat' or 'fertility') generally refers to the class of hormones produced by the body with similar oestrus-like actions. Chemicals with oestrogenic activity are produced naturally by many plants. Phyto-oestrogens refer to plant compounds with oestrogen-like activity, and mycoestrogens are produced by fungi. The three main groups of dietary phyto-oestrogens are isoflavones (enriched in soya beans, for example) coumestans (in clover and alfalfa sprouts) and lignans (oil seeds such as flax seeds).

Many scare stories about soya have appeared on the Internet, suggesting, for example, that it can shrink the brain or cause breast cancer. This does not even begin to pass the commonsense test when one remembers it has been a staple food for oriental people for at least four to five thousand years with no signs of such ill effects. Indeed, countries which use soya instead of dairy have the lowest rates of breast and prostate cancer in the world. Moreover, all of the reputable scientific papers we have read indicate that soya is protective against human breast and prostate cancer.[39] According to the Royal Society report on hormone-disrupting chemicals,[40] one of the beneficial ways in which plant oestrogens work is by reducing exposure of tissues to the body's own oestrogen. Plant oestrogens are found in almost all fruit and vegetables. Soya, lentils, peas and beans, which are legumes capable of fixing nitrogen from the air to make proteins, are a rich source of isoflavones. Typically oriental and Latin American diets include large quantities of legumes, and it has been calculated that a typical Western diet provides only about 3 mg of isoflavones a day compared with the 30 to 100 mg mg a day in the traditional oriental diet.

Red clover has particularly high levels of coumestans and, like chick peas (the basis of the Greek food hummus) and lentils, it contains all of the four important dietary isoflavones. Red clover, which can be bought from herbalists, is something Jane has started taking recently because she believes it to be protective against breast cancer. Sunflower seeds and alfalfa sprouts also contain substantial quantities of phyto-oestrogen compounds.

Phytoprogesterones in the diet may also be important in protecting against menopausal symptoms including osteoporosis. In his book *Natural Progesterone*,[41] Dr J. R. Lee argues that breast and other problems (including premenstrual tension, fibroids and weight gain, especially fat deposition at the hips and thighs) are caused by oestrogen dominance over progesterone, which can become worse as women approach the menopause. Dr Lee suggests that the problem is mainly the result of poor nutrition. He recommends including plenty of fresh vegetables, whole grains and fruit eaten as unprocessed as possible and uncontaminated by insecticides, artificial colouring agents or preservatives or other toxic ingredients. One of the richest sources of natural progesterone is wild yam or sweet potato, and soya and fennel contain both phyto-oestrogens and phytoprogesterones. Flax seed, because of its high content of lignans, which are converted in the digestive tract into substances that help to regulate endocrine function, has been shown in experiments to have a significant and specific role in sex steroid action by improving the progesterone/oestrogen ratio during menstrual cycles of women.[42] Much research on flax has been carried out by the US Food and Drug Administration, the National Cancer Institute and the Canadian Food Protection Branch.[43] The recommendation is to take about one tablespoon a day of flax seed in your diet for each 100 pounds of body weight (but be prepared to go to the loo more often!).

One of the most potent ways of using herbs (e.g. black cohosh, used by traditional Chinese medicine to treat menopausal symptoms) is to apply it as cream or patches. Wild yam cream (sometimes together with black cohosh) can be bought at most health shops and costs just a few pounds for a jar that lasts about six months.

Having had breast cancer five times, Jane has never been able to use hormone replacement therapy. Instead, she has a diet high in phytohormones. According to Dr J. R. Lee's wonderful book *Natural Progesterone*,[44] just adding soya to your diet a few times a week (although he recommends not to overdo this) can raise your bone density by as much as 6 per cent. Jane also uses a cream containing wild yam and black cohosh, both high in natural progesterone, and several of her friends including some well-known female scientists also swear by this cream. On a recent trip to Scotland Jane forgot to take her pot of cream with her and had no time to search out shops that sell it. She suffered from appalling hot flushes for the three days she was there and these symptoms were relieved only when she arrived home and applied her wild yam cream.

Dr Lee, controversially but convincingly, concludes that post-menopausal osteoporosis is a disease primarily of inadequate osteoblast-mediated new bone formation and he claims that natural progesterones applied to the skin using creams restore osteoblast function and are an essential factor in the prevention and proper treatment of osteoporosis. Dr Lee reported a 5–10 per cent increase in bone density in one year as a result of using natural progesterone cream, with no significant side effects.[45] We both strongly recommend that you read Dr Lee's book and consider his evidence, but DISCUSS HIS WORK AND FINDINGS WITH YOUR DOCTOR BEFORE MAKING ANY CHANGES IN YOUR MEDICAL REGIME.

The Desktop Guide to Complementary and Alternative Medicine: an evidence based approach,[46] which is generally considered an authoritative and comprehensive guide to the subject, surprisingly does not mention osteoporosis or wild yam. It states that 'there is no compelling evidence for the efficacy of any complementary treatment for alleviating menopausal symptoms, particularly in comparison with HRT. However, black cohosh looks encouraging in this respect and has a favourable safety profile . . . efforts to increase consumption of soya products may be worthwhile.' They report no known contraindications for any phyto-oestrogens, including soya, as part of the diet. Compare this with the risks associated with HRT.

LIFESTYLE FACTOR 6 EXERCISE

Bone loss with age cannot be explained entirely by declining physical activity levels.[47] If the bones are not loaded at all, as in space or during prolonged bedrest, however, they rapidly lose calcium, though the bones rapidly become remineralised when normal loading is restored.

Exercise has been proved in clinical trials to be helpful in the prevention and treatment of osteoporosis in both pre- and post-menopausal women.[48, 49] According to Lee,[50] weight-bearing exercise alone can stop the process of bone loss and add 1–2 per cent a year to bone mineral density.

Excessive exercise, on the other hand, causes microfractures in bones, which stimulates the osteoblasts to increase their activity – thus increasing their death rate.[51, 52] Excessive exercise causing stress in bones has been shown to be detrimental,[53, 54] though exercising specific muscles can be effective since strong muscles can absorb shock when falling.[55]

Normal activities are all the exercise needed to maintain bone health.

If you already have osteoporosis it is essential that any exercise plan is worked out with an appropriate health professional – your specialist consultant rheumatologist or orthopaedic doctor, or a qualified physiotherapist. According to

MedicineNet.com,[56] prudent exercise is important to avoid injury to already weakened bones. In patients over forty and in those with conditions such as heart disease, obesity, diabetes mellitus, high blood pressure, types and levels of exercise should be prescribed and monitored by their doctors.

Here are a few tips on exercise for those with the disease – and also for those at risk.[57, 58] Two of the most important types of exercise for bone health are weight-bearing and resistance exercise.

WEIGHT-BEARING EXERCISE

It is generally agreed that the best exercises for the bones are weight-bearing exercises (exercising against gravity). Examples include walking, jogging, dancing, stair-climbing, hiking, low-impact aerobics, tennis, golf and other outdoor games.

Avoid exercise that puts excessive stress on your bones, such as running or high-impact aerobics. Avoid rowing machines – they require deep forward bending that may lead to a vertebral fracture if you have fragile bones. Also avoid this exercise in general unless you have learned to do it with a professional trainer. It is one exercise that is particularly easy to get wrong. Extreme levels of exercise (such as marathon running) may not be healthy for the bones. Marathon running in young women that leads to weight loss and loss of menstrual periods can actually cause osteoporosis.

Swimming and stretching are not weight-bearing exercises and may not have a particularly beneficial effect on the bones.

All moderate outdoor exercise, including walking, is particularly beneficial because of the amount of vitamin D that will be formed by exposure of the skin to sunlight (even on a cloudy day). In contrast, lying around on a beach, covered with factor X sunblock cream, is not going to help your bones or your skin. If you must tan your body, do it the old-fashioned way by exposing your skin to sunshine very gradually, ideally while you are moving around outdoors.

According to Warren A. Katz and Carl Sherman,[59] brisk walking is an ideal exercise for most people who have osteoporosis. Walking can be done anywhere, requires no special equipment, costs nothing, and carries minimal risk of injury. If walking is too difficult or painful for you, workouts on a stationary exercise cycle are a good alternative.

The full benefits of walking come from a regular schedule – at least 15 to 20 minutes three to four days per week. But if you haven't been active for years, you may need to start modestly. Start at whatever level is comfortable for you. Five-minute walks are fine at first, but try increasing their length by one minute each day until you reach the optimal exercise level.

Walk briskly enough to become slightly short of breath. A little puffing shows that you're working your body hard enough to improve your fitness. If you have lung, heart, or other medical conditions, you should first consult your doctor about a safe level of activity. Also, the elderly who have impaired sight or hearing should be especially careful to avoid situations where they are likely to fall or have accidents – including traffic accidents.

RESISTANCE TRAINING

Lifting weights or using strength-training machines strengthens bones all over your body, especially if you exercise all of the major muscle groups in your legs, arms, and trunk. Following a programme designed by your doctor or a physical therapist is important. Joining a gym or fitness facility is a good way to begin because there you should have access to trainers who can advise you on proper technique.

Strength training is a slow process, so start at a low level and build up gradually over several months. For each exercise, select weights or set the machine so the muscle being trained becomes fatigued after ten to fifteen repetitions. As muscles strengthen, gradually add more weight. But don't increase the weight more than 10 per cent per week, since larger increases can raise your risk of injury. Remember to lift with good technique, and don't sacrifice good technique to lift more weight.

● Remember to lift and lower weights slowly to maximise muscle strength and minimise the risk of injury.
● It's best to perform your resistance workout every third day. This gives your body a chance to recover.

● Stiffness the morning after exercise is normal. But if you are in pain most of the following day, your joints are swollen, or you are limping, stop the programme until you are again comfortable, and cut your weights and repetitions by 25 per cent to 50 per cent. If bone, joint, or muscle pain is severe, call your doctor.

● If a particular area of your body feels sore immediately after exercise, apply ice for ten to fifteen minutes. Wrap ice in a towel, or just hold a cold can of juice to the spot.

● Vary your routine to make it more interesting. For example, if your strength-building programme involves twelve separate exercises, do six in one session and the other six in the next.

YOGA AND TAI-CHI

Yoga not only provides excellent exercise and body shaping: it also helps to calm the mind after a day's work. This is particularly helpful for those whose work involves using the brain more than the body. One of the great benefits of yoga is the breathing control that becomes second nature to users. This can help to keep blood CO_2 levels down, helping the body to eliminate one source of acid formed during metabolism.

Yoga is a particularly beneficial form of exercise, its main goal being to unite mind, body and spirit to enhance health and improve the quality of life. Indeed, yoga is a Sanskrit word meaning 'union'. It was developed by Hindu yogis at least 2,500 years ago. They believed that by following the six basic principles of yoga (proper exercise, proper breathing, adequate relaxation, proper diet, meditation and positive thinking) you can achieve total physical and mental health. Yoga is suitable for anyone of any age, and no special equipment or clothing is required. Many tapes, cassettes and books are available, but there is really no substitute for regular lessons with an experienced teacher. Meeting and talking with other people can also help to keep you motivated. There are several types of yoga, and you should try to become trained in the one most suitable for your age and physical fitness. Hatha yoga consists of gentle stretches with emphasis on developing a flexible spine. Sivananda yoga covers a wider range of poses, and emphasises diet and positive thinking. Vinaya yoga is the gentlest form of all, and is suitable for all ages, especially older people. Iyengar yoga and Ashtanga yoga are more physically challenging.

Tai-chi is a system of movement and postures rooted in ancient Chinese philosophy and martial arts used to enhance mental and physical health.[60] It is based on the two opposing life forces, yin and yang. The slow movement between different postures that are normally held for a short period of time are physical stimuli with effects on the cardiovascular and muscular systems. These stimuli, much like other physical exercise, result in increased muscle strength. In addition to adaptation processes, these effects can produce better co-ordination and balance. Thus tai-chi can help to decrease the risk of falling and, in turn, fracture,[61] including in the elderly. Ideally teachers should have had at least five years experience with a master.

ALEXANDER TECHNIQUE

It has been suggested[62] that the Alexander technique can help in osteoporosis by improving posture, mobility and safety. The technique was developed in the early part of the twentieth century by Frederick Alexander, an Australian actor who suffered recurring voice loss. By observing himself in the mirror he concluded that this was due to the tense position in which he usually held his head. By correcting the relationship between his head, neck and spine during activity, he solved the problem over a number of years. The Alexander technique is based on three principles:

● Function is affected by use
● An organism functions as a whole
● The relationship of the head, neck and spine is vital to optimum function

Certified teachers should have at least three years training on an approved course. According to Ernst,[63] the technique is almost entirely safe.

VIBRATING MACHINES

Preliminary data on more than fifty post-menopausal women[64] have shown that as little as twenty minutes a day on a vibrating platform can halt rapid bone loss. Newer data from a two-year study of sheep support this finding. It is believed that the vibrating platforms trigger bones to generate tiny electric fields that turn on the genes that effect bone remodelling and growth. These experimental anti-osteoporosis machines are just one example of new applications of electric and magnetic fields to bone disease and injures.

HORSES FOR COURSES

Gill has always been a keen sportswoman. She was captain of her school netball team and loved playing all sports. She is now a twelve-handicap golfer, who continues to win prizes.

In contrast, Jane has always disliked sport, so maintaining an exercise programme is particularly difficult for her. Even at school she avoided hockey, netball and tennis by hiding in a cellar under the changing rooms with others who did not like sport. However, she has always walked as much as possible, partly to arrive at interesting rocks and partly to avoid waiting for buses or underground trains for short journeys. She now makes a point of MBWA (management by walking about), rather than sitting at her computer all day using e-mail to make contact with staff and colleagues. She finds this not only keeps her healthy, it also improves relationships. She sometimes wears a pedometer (these can be purchased from good sports-equipment shops) to check that she does at least 5,000 steps a day. On a recent shopping trip to town one of her friends did 15,000 steps, so retail therapy is fine.

We have both joined a gym and Jane works hard to defeat the boredom she feels by taking interesting tapes to play on her walkman or by deliberately devising ideas for research or chapters for her books. The exercise regimen she finds most helpful, however, is yoga.

LIFESTYLE FACTOR 7 AVOIDING FALLS AND FRACTURES

This applies especially to people who already suffer from osteoporosis.

The US National Institute of Health, Osteoporosis, website gives the following valuable advice to osteoporosis sufferers on how to avoid falls.[65]

Fall Prevention is a special concern for men and women with osteoporosis. Falls can increase the likelihood of fracturing a bone in the hip, wrist, spine or other part of the skeleton. In addition to the environmental factors listed below, falls can also be caused by impaired vision and/or balance, chronic diseases that impair mental or physical functioning, and certain medications, such as sedatives and antidepressants. It is important that individuals with osteoporosis be aware of any physical changes they may be experiencing that affect their balance or gait, and that they discuss these changes with their health care provider.

Some tips to help eliminate the environmental factors that lead to falls include:

Outdoors. Use a cane or walker for added stability; wear rubber-soled shoes for traction; walk on grass when pavements are slippery; in winter, carry salt or kitty litter to sprinkle on slippery pavements; be careful on highly polished surfaces that become slippery and dangerous when wet.

Indoors. Keep rooms free of clutter, especially on floors; keep floor surfaces smooth but not slippery; wear supportive, low-heeled shoes even at home; avoid walking in socks, stockings, or slippers; be sure carpets and rugs have skid-proof backing or are tacked to the floor; be sure stairwells are well lit and that stairs have handrails on both sides; install grab bars on bathroom walls near the bath, shower, and toilet; use a rubber bath mat in shower or bath; keep a torch with fresh batteries beside your bed; if using a step stool for hard to reach areas, use a sturdy one with a handrail and wide steps. Consider purchasing a cordless phone so that you don't have to rush to answer the phone when it rings or you can call for help if you do fall.

Many simple, objective measures of frailty can help to assess the risk of fracture. These include the ability to rise from a chair without use of the arms, depth perception, contrast sensitivity, and gait and balance assessment.[66]

Hip protectors are devices that reduce the likelihood of a hip fracture in a fall. A pad or shield is held in place over the hip. Many types of device are marketed around the world and they fit into two main types. The first rely on pads made of an energy-absorbing material, while the second uses a semi-rigid plastic shield to divert force from the hip to the soft tissues of the thigh. The first large-scale randomised trial of hip protectors, in 1991, showed a 56 per cent risk reduction through use. Another recently published large-scale trial has reported broadly similar conclusions. Hip protectors are mainly available for women, but are now being manufactured also for men. Many clinical trials of such devices are in progress, and one has found that people

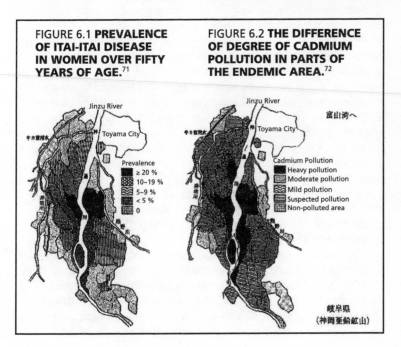

FIGURE 6.1 **PREVALENCE OF ITAI-ITAI DISEASE IN WOMEN OVER FIFTY YEARS OF AGE.**[71]

FIGURE 6.2 **THE DIFFERENCE OF DEGREE OF CADMIUM POLLUTION IN PARTS OF THE ENDEMIC AREA.**[72]

who use them feel more confident that they can avoid injury by wearing them.[67]

LIFESTYLE FACTOR 8 POLLUTION

CADMIUM

The strange disease that appeared in the downstream basin of the Jinzu River, Toyana, in west-central Japan around 1912[68] was called by locals 'Itai-Itai byo' ('itai' is what Japanese people say when in severe pain, just as Westerners say 'ouch', and 'byo' literally means disease). It came by this name because of the way victims cried out 'Itai-Itai' as a result of the excruciating pain they suffered. It was mostly post-menopausal women who were afflicted, sometimes with pain across their entire body. In the most severe cases, they suffered broken bones when simply trying to move around on their own. However, because the disease was first taken as an endemic sickness, it wasn't until the 1950s that meaningful research began.

In 1956, a local general medical practitioner, Dr Hagino, announced his opinion that Itai-Itai disease was a form of bone brittleness that came about as a result of malnutrition. Later, however, when he noted that the outbreak was concentrated in a particular area of the Jinzu River basin, he announced that the disease was due to cadmium poisoning caused by high concentrations of this heavy metal carried in the Jinzu River.

Just as Dr Snow (see page 13) used simple plots to identify the Broad Street pump as the cause of the cholera epidemic in London in September 1854,[69] Dr Hagino used the same type of epidemiological evidence to show the strong correlation between the prevalence of Itai-Itai disease in women over fifty years of age and the degree of cadmium pollution.[70] The degree of cadmium pollution in different parts of the endemic area determined by the analysed cadmium concentration of the soil in the paddy fields is shown in Figure 6.2. In Figure 6.1, the frequency of the disease is illustrated by the percentage of women over fifty years of age having or suspected of having the disease. The correlation between the prevalence of Itai-Itai disease and the degree of cadmium pollution was striking.

Animal studies on the effect of cadmium on bone formation[73] show that it inhibits osteoblasts in bone marrow through direct effects on these cells.

In May 1968, a full twelve years after Dr Hagino's brilliant discovery, the Japanese Ministry of Health and Welfare officially announced that Itai-Itai disease was chronic cadmium poisoning, first impairing kidney function and progressively causing bone disease. Victims suffer from calcium deficiency as occurs with old age, malnutrition and hormone imbalance. The report concluded that the cadmium came from discharges from the operation of base-metal mines into the Jinzu River. (The world's leading modern mining companies now go to great lengths to prevent any toxic discharges to the environment.)

Cadmium is a toxic heavy metal that accumulates in the body and has a slow elimination half life of twenty to thirty years.[74] It is stored in the kidney and at high levels produces damage to the proximal kidney tubule. Most non-exposed people, those without known exposure, have kidney concentrations below 30 mcg/g.[75] Cigarette smoking doubles the kidney concentration in smokers and is so overwhelming that it is a confounding factor in epidemiologic studies looking at other types of exposure. A variety of low-molecular-weight proteins which are normally present at very low levels in the urine are elevated in the urine of cadmium-exposed people, due to the tubular damage which inhibits the normal process of reabsorption. Cadmium may also cause anaemia, teeth discoloration (from the formation of cadmium sulphide) and loss of sense of smell.

According to the US Occupational Safety and Health Administration,[76] most exposure to cadmium is in industrial workplaces, particularly where metal ore is being processed or smelted.

Major sources of pollution potentially affecting the population at large include the application of sewage sludge and compost, the use of fertilisers based on certain types of rock phosphate, waste incineration, and fossil fuel combustion. The British Geological Survey and the Soil Survey have published maps showing cadmium levels over the UK. The Environment Agency may be able to tell you of any particular problems in your area. Such information is usually available from similar national surveys and agencies in other countries.

FLUORIDE

Although fluoride is generally regarded as essential, there is no evidence from human studies that overt clinical signs of fluoride deficiency exist.[77] Fluoride has a complex and frequently indirect relationship with susceptibility to dental caries[78] (tooth decay). Animal experiments suggest it may be a structurally important constituent of bone collagen and the vascular system. Fluoride can be extremely toxic, however, and the level of intake compatible with human health is extremely low. Dental mottling may be taken as an early definitive indication of toxicity. Long-term exposure to high levels of fluoride leads to destruction of the teeth. Fluoride is a cumulative toxin, most being trapped by bone tissue where it locally stimulates new bone formation. Bone outgrowth caused in this way can give rise to considerable ill health, including heart and nerve diseases, and high fluoride also interferes with collagen synthesis in bone. In toxic amounts, fluoride interferes with calcium metabolism; increased bone accretion rate, increased bone resorption rate and increased total body turnover of calcium have all been reported. Ingestion of large amounts of fluoride (5–40 mg per day) in drinking water causes kyphosis, spine and joint deformities, and dramatic skeletal deformity in areas of Iran, Kenya and Tanzania. The symptoms of fluoride toxicity include osteoporosis.[79] The problem tends to be most serious in soft water areas because hard water contains calcium which removes fluorine from the water. It has been suggested that adult intakes in excess of 5 mg of fluoride per day from all sources pose a significant risk of skeletal fluorosis. According to Lee,[80] fluoride is a potent enzyme inhibitor and causes pathological changes in bone, leading to increased risk of fracture. He recommends that fluoride in all forms, including toothpaste, be avoided.

Although fluoride may be necessary, in tiny amounts, to prevent dental caries, the information from WHO[81] suggests that, as a society, we are using far too much fluoride.

ALUMINIUM

Aluminium can adversely affect health,[82] including that of the bones and skeleton if consumption is excessive since it markedly reduces bone formation. Aluminium in excess can reduce the absorption of calcium, magnesium and phosphorus.[83] In the past, people undergoing dialysis were affected by excess aluminium which markedly reduced their bone formation. Aluminium interacts with several other elements, including calcium, fluorine, iron, magnesium, phosphorus and strontium, and when ingested can reduce their absorption.

Exposure to aluminium has increased as production has gone up rapidly in the twentieth century, with about 15 million tons per year being produced by the early 1980s. Human exposure to aluminium may also have increased since both the solubility and bioavailability to plants and aquatic life of environmental aluminium may have been increased by acid rain. Normal Western diets are not considered to pose a problem except in people with impaired kidney function. Water can supply from less than 100 mcg to 1 mg per litre depending on how acid it is, with higher aluminium in more acid waters such as those draining upland peat areas. The use of aluminium cooking utensils with acid foods may increase intake. According to the WHO,[84] milk, milk products and cereal products typically account for about 60 per cent of total dietary intake of aluminium. The most important contribution to aluminium intake, however, can be from antacid medications, some of which provide several grams of the metal per day! These amounts interfere with the absorption of other elements important to the skeleton (see above) and also may lead to a gradual accumulation of aluminium in the skeleton.

TIN

Tin toxicity has been shown to interfere with the metabolism of calcium, copper and zinc – all essential to healthy bones.[85] The main dietary intake of tin is from canned food. Toxicity from tin is normally associated with food contaminated by corrosion of tin-lined cans.

HORMONE-DISRUPTING CHEMICALS

When we began writing this section it did not occur to us to suggest that bone disease might be promoted by some of the chemicals discussed in *Your Life in Your Hands*,[86] because these are known to be predominantly fat-soluble and to accumulate in fatty tissue such as the breast. Recently, however, we have become aware of research into the way in which bone marrow and the surrounding bone, with its high storage capacity for inorganic chemicals such as fluoride and radioactive elements, may also accumulate chemicals such as benzene and its metabolites.[87] Also, the hormone-disrupting substances may affect how the sex hormones, including oestrogen and the thyroid hormones, behave.[88] Hence, limiting our exposure to them may help, directly or indirectly, to reduce bone disease. The three groups of most concern are the oestrogens, anti-androgens and thyroid hormone disrupters. Hormone-disrupting chemicals are of particular concern because they can interfere with the normal function of the hormonal (chemical messenger) system of the body. Such properties are found in several classes of chemicals released into the environment, such as some insecticides and fungicides and some phthalate plasticisers used to make plastics soft and bendy – including some used to wrap foods. There is controversy about the effect of these chemicals on humans, but it is generally accepted that a biocide called tributyl tin caused populations of molluscs such as dog whelks and oysters to be wiped out around southern Britain in the 1970s because the females developed male organs which blocked their egg tubes, causing death. The case of sites on UK rivers where 100 per cent of the fish are intersex fish (with the characteristics of both sexes), especially downstream of sewage works, has highlighted the fact that a wide range of chemicals in the environment may exert such an effect.[89, 90, 91]

It was more than twenty years ago that sexual disruption in fish was first reported in the UK by Thames Water Authority staff acting on casual observations by anglers.[92] Their findings were filed as an internal report, and no further action was taken. In the mid-1980s, effluents from sewage-treatment works discharging into rivers in England and Wales were found to be oestrogenic, due to their ability to induce the production of female characteristics in male fish. In some rivers the main cause is thought to be substances called alkyl pherols (from detergents); in many other rivers it is thought to be residues from the female contraceptive pill which contains synthetic oestrogen, which is much more potent than natural oestrogen, together with natural oestrogen.

There is further discussion of these chemicals in *Your Life in Your Hands*[93] and in various other sources including *Our Stolen Futures* by Colborn, Dumanski and Myers. We are not going to repeat the discussion here. We are, however, going to give you some advice on how to limit your exposure to damaging chemicals in the environment as much as possible, based on the advice given in *Your Life in Your Hands*.

AVOIDING HARMFUL SUBSTANCES IN THE ENVIRONMENT – PRACTICALITIES

SMOKING

One of the main sources of pollutants to try to eliminate is tobacco smoking. The link between smoking and lung cancer is well known, and it is also implicated in cancer of the mouth, windpipe, oesophagus, bladder and pancreas. It is estimated that smoking tobacco causes approximately 30 per cent of all cancers in the USA. Tobacco smoke is of particular concern in protecting bones from damage because of its effect on female hormones and its content of cadmium (see page 125).

Cadmium concentrations increase with age, even in the general population. However, most non-exposed people have kidney concentrations below 30 mcg/g. Cigarette smoking is a potent source of cadmium, doubling the kidney concentration in smokers and confounding epidemiologic studies (see page 125). A variety of low molecular weight proteins which are normally present at very low levels in the urine, are elevated in the urine of cadmium-exposed people, due to the tubular damage which inhibits the normal process of reabsorption. These biomarkers are elevated in those exposed to cadmium.

If you do smoke and are addicted to nicotine and find it difficult to give up, you can reduce your risks of bone disease, cancer, heart disease and stroke by having the nicotine as patches or by chewing nicotine-impregnated gum, because it is the tar and other contaminants in tobacco smoke that contain the health-damaging agents, not the nicotine. Such is the power of advertising and image that young people – including, increasingly, young women – are persuaded to spend a lot of money taking up smoking, a habit which makes them progressively less attractive to the rest of us to look at and smell.

WATER SUPPLY

In much of the Western world, especially cities, dwellers are likely to drink water that is recycled surface water after treatment in sewage works – we often joke that in the East End of London the water has been drunk by about fifteen people before us. According to the Royal Society report on endocrine (hormone) disrupting chemicals,[94] synthetic oestrogens such as DES, hexestrol and ethinyl oestradiol used in oral contraception and HRT find their way into river water, and 'very low levels may occur in some drinking water'. While drinking water must meet stringent criteria, we prefer to reduce our risk of being exposed to damaging chemicals (including residues from the female contraceptive pill, other pharmaceuticals or their residues, fertiliser and pesticide residues, and hormone-disrupting chemicals generally) by filtering our water. We simply use a filter system with a glass jug and replace the cartridge according to the manufacturer's instructions. Boiling water before use causes further breakdown of some pollutants. Unfortunately filtering and boiling water also reduces levels of calcium and magnesium. We limit our use of bottled water, some of which contains levels of pollutants that would be illegal in tap water. We particularly avoid water stored in plastic bottles.

MAN-MADE CHEMICALS: SOME TIPS ON HOW TO LIMIT YOUR EXPOSURE TO THEM

Most supermarkets now have a good range of organically produced food, and one can also find local suppliers over the

Internet. In the case of clothes, furnishings, personal care products and toys, some retailers are systematically phasing out hazardous chemicals from their products. In the UK, these retailers include Boots, B&Q, the Co-op, the Early Learning Centre, Homebase and Marks and Spencer.[95] Here is a list of some of the things you can do to limit your exposure to man-made chemicals:

● Eat organically produced food, which uses far less and far fewer chemical pesticides and fertilisers. Sewage sludge application is prohibited by the Soil Association and the amount of cadmium allowed in rock phosphate fertiliser is prescribed.

● If you must use make-up use hypoallergenic ranges, which generally contain fewer preservatives and other potential chemical sensitisers. The label on some expensive shower gel marketed by a prestigious company actually lists phthalates – one of the main groups of endocrine disrupters implicated in the feminisation of fish – among the chemicals it contains. Research by Professor John Sumpter of Brunel University, London, now suggests that parabens (a very common preservative in cosmetics) could be an oestrogen-mimic (hormone-disrupting chemical – see page 128).[96] With cosmetics, as with all other products: read the label, and remember – simpler is better.

● Do not wear perfume, and use simple, unperfumed soap and deodorants.

● Do not add chemicals other than simple salts such as Epsom salts to your bath water.

● Avoid fluoride toothpaste and mouth washes. There are good non-fluoride toothpastes – and even common salt or baking soda will do a good job of cleaning your teeth. In any case, always rinse your mouth very thoroughly after cleaning your teeth.

● Try to use cars as little as possible, and walk or travel by public transport instead. The chemicals emitted by cars, even when well tuned and running optimally, include many hazardous substances such as benzene (see John Pearson's book *The Air Quality Challenge*[97]).

● If you paint your house or have it painted, ensure it is well ventilated (some of the oil-based paints used in Britain are now banned in Scandinavia). Also, new furniture, curtains and upholstery can be important sources of formaldehyde, brominated flame retardents and benzene, and benzene is given off by many fast-drying glues. Polyvinyl chlorides (PVCs) should also be avoided as much as possible. In an article in *The Times* of 11 November 1999 by Martin Fletcher, it was reported that the European Commission had called for an emergency ban on soft PVC (polyvinyl chloride) toys, including rattles and dummies which babies suck. It is claimed that these contain dangerous chemicals. Again, the dangerous chemicals concerned are phthalates. Use wood, glass, ceramics and natural mineral materials in the home, and stainless steel, enamel or toughened glass for cooking and aluminium foil to wrap food. Use natural materials for furnishing whenever you can, with as few plastics or man-made fibres or other chemicals as possible.

● Limit your use of chemicals in the garden. If some plant in the garden is going to die, so be it. Feed it with composted household waste to help it survive but minimise your use of chemicals in the garden. Our gardens have lots of different wild bird species, butterflies, ladybirds, toads and hedgehogs. The degree of biodiversity in our gardens compared to those of many friends who use chemicals says a great deal about the damage the use of chemicals does to the animals – so why do we think that we will be unaffected?

● Never use aerosol sprays for hair, deodorants, cleaning, gardening or any other purpose because of the increased risk of inhaling synthetic chemicals.

● Use natural materials for clothing wherever possible. Always wash and thoroughly rinse new clothes before wearing them, to remove preservatives.

● When washing crockery and cutlery, minimise the use of detergents and ensure that they are thoroughly rinsed off before use.

● Recycle paper, glass, metals, plastics, clothes and books, and be especially careful in the appropriate recycling of any batteries that could contain cadmium or other metals.

You might find it strange that someone like Jane, who has spent her professional career working in chemical laboratories, should try so hard to avoid chemicals in everyday life. Like many of her colleagues, she has a healthy respect for what chemicals can do to biological processes – and so minimises her exposure.

If you have good, nutritious food and reduce exposure to pollutants, you will find your skin and general appearance improve without the need to add polluting man-made chemicals to your body or the environment. We can all reduce our personal risk from hazardous chemicals and by doing so we help the environment generally, with cleaner water and soils and hence more wholesome food. To most natural scientists this is all just common sense and is very easy to live with.

It is impossible to eliminate risk entirely from man-made chemical substances, but you can reduce your personal risk by following the guidelines above and whenever you read or hear a new advertisement for a new beauty product, man-made fabric or garden spray, for example, think very carefully whether you really need it. Almost certainly you do not.

7 'It's an Ill Wind that Blows No One any Good'

from John Heywood's 1546 proverb collection

In this chapter we look first at some of the appalling human and social costs of osteoporosis in countries such as the USA, Canada and the UK. We then examine the implications of the disease being treated (ludicrously) as one of dietary calcium deficiency. Finally, we consider some of the vested-interest groups and organisations that are profiting from the toll the disease is taking. These range from the dairy industry and calcium and vitamin manufacturers and retailers to the manufacturers of diagnostic equipment and pharmaceuticals to treat the disease. We end with ten golden guidelines for you to follow.

In *Your Life in Your Hands*, the concluding chapter pointed out that all the information, epidemiology, scientific experiments and research that Jane had pieced together had all been published in the scientific literature. Some of this information had been available for years, evense decades. It was just that Jane had never heard of it, despite reading good newspapers and respected scientific journals such as *Nature* and *New Scientist*. Jane therefore asked, 'Why have we not been told about it?' She concluded that all the pieces of the jigsaw had been there in the scientific literature, but because of the way that science is now funded, particularly its increasing privatisation, nobody had put the pieces together.

We cannot ask the same question in this book, because many other scientists and doctors have reached the same conclusions as we have and published them in books, magazine articles and a multitude of websites, as we shall see. We are forced to conclude that orthodox medicine and national and international agencies and charities are literally feeding us the wrong message, but this time we must ask why they have not taken account of the widely publicised information about the principal causes of osteoporosis. Let us look more closely at what is happening, first of all by looking at the devastation the ill wind is causing.

THE ILL WIND

According to the US National Institutes of Health, osteoporosis is a major public health threat for 28 million Americans,[1] 80 per cent of whom are women. In the US today 10 million individuals have osteoporosis and 18 million more have low bone mass (according to the WHO criteria), placing them at increased risk of the disease. It is estimated that one out of every two women and one in eight men over fifty there will have an osteoporosis-related fracture in their lifetime. More than 2 million American men already suffer from osteoporosis, and millions more are at risk. Each year, 80,000 men suffer a hip fracture and one third of these men die within a year. However, osteoporosis can strike at any age. Osteoporosis is responsible for more than 1.5 million fractures annually, including 300,000 hip fractures, and approximately 700,000 vertebral fractures, 250,000 wrist fractures, and more than 300,000 fractures at other sites.

Complications of osteoporosis are a major community health problem in terms of both social and healthcare costs. The estimated cost of fractures caused by osteoporosis in 1995 in the USA was a staggering $13.8 billion.[2] Most of this money ($10.3 billion, or 75 per cent) was spent on the treatment of fractures in white women.[3] These investigations[4, 5] confirmed the well-recognised observation that osteoporosis is principally a problem of ageing white women. Nevertheless, 23 per cent of healthcare expenditure for the disease was incurred by white men (18 per cent) and non-white women (5 per cent). Even the group least susceptible to osteoporotic fracture in the USA, non-white men, cost $200 million in osteoporosis care in 1995.[6] Most of this money (63 per cent) was spent on caring for those with hip fractures, the remaining 37 per cent being spent on other types of fractures.[7] While every effort was made to capture relevant data, fractures other than hip fractures were probably under-reported, because most of them do not require hospital admission.

In Canada, 1.4 million people suffer from osteoporosis.[8] One in four women there over the age of fifty has the condition, and one in eight men over fifty. The cost of treating osteoporosis and the fractures it causes is estimated to be $1.3 billion each year. Long-term, hospital and chronic care account for most of these costs. Without effective action on osteoporosis prevention and treatment strategies, it is estimated that over the next 25 years Canada will spend at least $32.5 billion treating osteoporotic fractures. Given the increasing proportion of older people in the population, these costs are likely to rise.

The statistics related to hip fracture there are particularly disturbing. There are approximately 25,000 hip fractures each year, 70 per cent of which are osteoporosis-related. Hip fractures result in death in 20 per cent of cases and disability in 50 per cent of those that survive. More women in Canada die each year of osteoporotic fractures than from breast and ovarian cancer combined.

In the UK, 22.5 per cent of women over the age of fifty suffer from osteoporosis. The majority (60,000) suffer with hip problems and over 40,000 from problems relating to the spinal vertebrae. 20 per cent of all hip fractures result in death, 50 per cent end up with impaired mobility and a further 20 per cent lose their independence as a result.[9]

In England and Wales the cost of osteoporotic fractures in 1990 was estimated to be £742 million per year.[10] Osteoporosis is now known to cost £750 million a year of which 33 per cent is spent on acute injuries resulting from the condition and the remaining 66 per cent is spent on rehabilitation and community care.[11]

It is clear that osteoporosis and associated fractures are a major public health concern because they account for a significant amount of serious illness, disability, diminished quality of life and, in the most serious cases, death. The cost of care is high, and the implications for public-health expenditure are serious if effective action is not taken.

There are human costs in addition to the financial costs.[12] The reduced quality of life for those with osteoporosis is enormous. Osteoporosis can result in disfigurement, lowered self-esteem, reduction or loss of mobility, and decreased independence.

Is it possible that this situation is benefiting anyone – or, worse, that it is being exploited to make profits by vested interest groups? Let us look at some of the possibilities.

CASH COWS

Throughout most of Western society milk is promoted as a healthy, wholesome, natural food: vital for babies, full of protein for growth and health, a slimming drink for the young wanting to look their best and, above all now, as an essential source of calcium for women at risk of osteoporosis. The simple-minded approach that even many medical professionals appear to have taken on board is: in osteoporosis the bone degenerates – the bone needs lots of calcium – milk and cheese contain lots of calcium – so if you have lots of milk and cheese all will be well. The widely publicised scientific evidence on the real causes of osteoporosis appears to have made no impact on conventional thinking. We have been unable to find a single website from an orthodox medical source, national or international agency or charity that does not recommend dairy as a source of calcium and protection against osteoporosis.

Looking at the websites of major international organisations and charities dedicated to osteoporosis which, as far as we can see, all push the high-calcium and calcium-equals-dairy myth, one is left wondering why they do not know or will not acknowledge the overwhelming evidence against the Western diet, with its high dependency on dairy produce and other animal protein. Why all this support for the calcium myth when the epidemiological (at the global and local scales) physiological, biochemical and nutritional scientific evidence from peer-reviewed literature all points overwhelmingly to the problem being a diet too high in animal protein – cheese being the worst offender – and too low in vegetable foods.

Let us quote, as an example, from the website of the main international osteoporosis organisation:

The International Osteoporosis Foundation (IOF) is an international non-governmental organization whose bylaws were registered in Berne, Switzerland in 1987 as the European Foundation for Osteoporosis (EFFO). In 1998, EFFO joined forces with the International Federation of Societies on Skeletal Diseases (IFSSD), established 1995. IOF's **mission** is to advance the understanding of **osteoporosis** and to promote prevention, diagnosis and treatment of the disease worldwide.

The Foundation is composed of:
- a **Committee of 138 National Societies** representing 71 countries
- a **Committee of Scientific Advisors** comprising 68 members
- a **Committee of Corporate Advisors** representing 33 companies

The organization is managed by a **Board** which delegates day-to-day responsibility to an **Executive Committee**, and **staff members** with input from the above committees.[13]

The IOF's position statement on milk products and osteoporosis contains the following summary:

Milk and milk products are valuable and usually well-tolerated sources of natural calcium which can help to prevent osteoporosis. It is disturbing that dogmatic arguments are used to blame a nutrient which is important for a healthy diet.[14]

The author of this summary statement on milk is the Board member for Germany, Professor Helmut W. Minne. Does he not know that his country has one of the highest, if not the highest, rates of osteoporosis in the world? So why should anyone listen to this advice from him?

We repeat: **the countries and communities with the lowest dairy consumption have incredibly low bone fracture rates compared with countries such as Germany and the USA where approximately 40 per cent of the diet consists of**

dairy produce, and there are good physiological reasons to explain this as we have discussed in Chapters 3 and 4.

Let us quote from John Robbins's best-selling book *Diet for a New America*[15] – a book which was first published as long ago as 1987:

> I used to believe that bones lost calcium only if there were not enough calcium in our diets. The [US] National Dairy Council is the foremost spokesman for this point of view and the solution they propose not all that surprisingly is for us all to drink more milk and eat more dairy products. In fact the dairy industry has of late spent a great deal of money promoting this point of view, and it does seem logical. But nutritional research clearly indicates a major flaw in this perspective. Osteoporosis is caused by a number of things the most important of which is excess dietary protein!

Robbins goes on to say:
> The [US] National Dairy Council has spent tens of millions of dollars to make us think that osteoporosis can be prevented by drinking more milk and eating more dairy products. But the only research that even begins to suggest that the consumption of dairy products might be helpful has been paid for by the National Dairy Council itself.

The same point about the dairy industry funding of research has been made by Dr R. D. Kradjian MD, the Chief of the Breast Surgery Division at the Seton Medical Centre, Daly City, California in his book *Save Yourself from Breast Cancer*[16] and in a letter entitled 'The Milk Letter: A Message to my Patients'.[17]

Let us also quote from Dr John McDougall MD, a leading medical authority on dietary associations with disease:

> **The myth that osteoporosis is caused by calcium deficiency was created to sell dairy products and calcium supplements.** There's no truth to it. American women are among the biggest consumers of calcium in the world, and

they still have one of the highest levels of osteoporosis in the world. And eating even more dairy products and calcium supplements is not going to change that fact.[18]

McDougall concludes[19]

The primary cause of osteoporosis is the high-protein diet most Americans consume today. As one leading researcher in this area said, 'Eating a high-protein diet is like pouring acid rain on your bones.'

Perhaps the most disturbing point McDougall makes, and one with which we agree after examining available nutritional studies and evidence, is the following:

I would like to emphasise that the calcium-losing effects of protein in the human body is not an area of controversy in scientific circles. The many studies performed during the past 55 years consistently show that the most important dietary change that we can make if we want to create a positive calcium balance that will keep our bones solid is to decrease the amount of protein we eat each day.[20]

It has also been said that[21]

Remarkably enough, if dairy has any effect, both clinical and population evidence strongly implicate dairy in causing, rather than preventing, osteoporosis. **That the dairy industry would lull unsuspecting women and children into complacency by telling them, essentially, drink more milk and your bones will be fine, may make good business sense, but it does the public a grave disservice.**

There are many other problems with consuming dairy produce, which has been linked to breast and prostate cancer,[22, 23, 24, 25] to colic, sickness and anaemia in babies fed on cow's milk.[26, 27, 28, 29, 30] Infants can develop facial or generalised eczema, persistent nasal congestion and noisy wheezing with or without gastrointestinal disturbance.[31] Milk is the single most common cause of allergy in infants.[32]

The late Dr Benjamin Spock, in *Baby and Child Care* (the United States' best selling book, other than the Bible, over the past fifty years), after recommending that no one consume cow's milk and cataloguing a host of ills associated with milk consumption (heart disease, cancer, obesity, antibiotic residue, iron deficiency, asthma, ear infections, skin conditions, stomach aches, bloating and diarrhoea), concludes: 'In nature, animals do not drink milk after infancy, and that is the normal pattern for humans, too . . . Children stay in better calcium balance when their protein comes from plant sources.' Dr Spock recommends human mother's milk for baby humans, as nature intended.

Insulin-dependent diabetes (Type 1 or childhood-onset) has been linked to dairy products.[33] The intensive dairy industry is also important in the transmission of infectious disease, including Johne's disease in cows. This disease is believed to be associated with irritable bowel syndrome in humans,[34] which affects 20 per cent of the population in the USA.[35] Listeria monocytogenes, which can cause meningitis and septicaemia, especially in vulnerable people such as infants, the elderly and the immunosuppressed, is a bacterium which can occur in soft cheeses.[36] Bovine tuberculosis can also infect humans, as can brucellosis, leptospirosis (Weil's disease) and cryptosporidium, which is a malaria-like parasite resistant to normal water disinfection processes that is even affecting our major underground water sources. The dairy industry contributes to the spread of all these diseases, not to mention BSE and new-variant CJD. Even in the European Union, which has high regulatory standards, milk for human consumption can be sold legally when levels of pus cells in it are so high that a 5 ml teaspoon can contain 2 million of them. To quote from the *Sunday Times*, 'In reality, the modern high-yield dairy cow is a pitiful ramshackle embodiment of market-driven exploitation. The new UK model, so help us, is the American holstein battery cow. A shed-housed fermentation vat on legs, teats dragging on the ground, it's a sight to frighten children'.[37] The article includes a photograph of 'a large-uddered milker, one of the grotesque products of the modern dairy industry'. The article goes on to point out that farmers have not been able to resist the genetic promise (of developing such creatures) – a 2 per cent compound increase in milk yield annually. Referring to osteoporosis, the *Sunday Times* article states:

> As The American Journal of Clinical Nutrition recently concluded, 'Age-related bone loss may be more attributable to *excess calcium loss* than to *inadequate calcium intake*'. [Our italics.]
>
> That's the bone breaker: excess calcium loss. Where the dairy industry and public policy get it wrong is in placing undue importance on calcium intake. For one thing, other dietary factors operate like bone thieves. Salt and animal protein . . . all result in net calcium losses through urine. Conversely, extra potassium from a diet rich in fruit and vegetables buttresses retained calcium by limiting losses. Walsh [Dr Stephen Walsh, Lecturer in Advanced Process Control at Imperial College, London] puts it well: 'Relying on calcium alone to prevent osteoporosis is like fielding a football team with only strikers and no defenders'.
>
> The critical factor, then, is calcium balance – and on that score, the white stuff falls down badly. Several substances in milk, particularly protein, contribute to calcium losses. Result: a third of the calcium initially absorbed by the body from milk is then wasted, through urine, in losses caused by the milk itself; from cheese, more than two-thirds is wasted. Bad news for those with poor calcium absorption, as among many elderly people and the genetically prone.
>
> So which are the best foods? Granny was right: eat your greens!

FRUITFUL ORGANIC ARGUMENTS

It is unfortunate in the UK that the Food Standards Agency and the Advertising Standards Agency do not pursue the claims of the Dairy Council with the same vigour that they have applied against the organic food producers. Let us once again quote from the *Sunday Times* article:

'Taken all together – the welfare and environmental issues, and the adverse health evidence – it points to a fundamental change in British agriculture', says Rayner [Dr Mike Rayner, a nutrition and heart specialist at Oxford University]. 'But there's huge reluctance on the part of the farming community, and the Food Standards Agency doesn't even have it on its agenda to move us away from an animal-dependent system to a more plant-based agriculture. It makes no sense.'

FALSE CLAIMS[38]

Last year [2001], in an attempt to clamp down on false and misleading claims, the Advertising Standards Authority (ASA) issued guidelines for advertisers on claims about organic food. This was prompted by several complaints received by the ASA about organic claims made by well-known names, including Tesco and the Soil Association. The new guidelines state that:

● Advertisers can't claim that organic food is 'safer' or 'healthier' than conventional food, unless they have convincing evidence that this is the case.

● Organic food can't be described as 'environmentally friendly' or 'sustainable', as all managed food production systems cause some environmental damage.

● Claims that organic food uses no chemicals, pesticides or artificial additives can only be made if this is the case.

In Chapter 6 we have argued that one of the best ways of limiting the ingestion of toxic man-made substances is by eating organically grown food, ideally produced locally to standards such as those of the Soil Association.

An article in *Which?* magazine[39] discusses the advantages of organically produced food:

One of the most common reasons our shoppers gave for choosing organic food was to avoid pesticides. Organic standards allow the use of some approved pesticides but these are mostly from natural sources. There's little data on pesticide residue levels in organic food, but the government's pesticide residue monitoring programme (see *Which?*, September 2001, p24) includes a limited number of organic samples, and residues are rarely found in those tested . . . Processing can significantly reduce the levels of residues. Washing and peeling alone has been shown to reduce levels by 50 to 90 per cent in apples, carrots and potatoes. Cooking and other types of processing involving heat can reduce levels further . . .

Organic food production emphasises environmental protection – for example, it aims to enhance biological diversity and maintain long-term soil fertility. Also, by restricting the use of artificial fertilisers and pesticides, organic farmers and agricultural workers reduce the risk of harmful health effects to themselves as well as the risk of environmental damage associated with more intensive pesticide use.

But there are also less favourable environmental considerations concerning organic processed food. Around 70 per cent of organic food is imported to the UK. This has its own environmental impact in terms of transport, packaging, waste and pollution. One way round this is to buy locally produced organic food. Food processing also has environmental costs in terms of energy use and packaging . . .

Organic food can contain food additives (E numbers) and processing aids, but the list is more restricted – around 35 additives are approved, compared with hundreds in conventional food. Artificial sweeteners are banned and only natural flavourings and colourings are allowed . . .

At least 95 per cent of the agricultural ingredients must be organic, and the other 5 per cent can be made up of non-organic ingredients, such as approved herbs and spices. Non-agricultural ingredients such as water, salt and additives approved for use in organic food are not included in these calculations . . .

Ideally, organic animals are given purely organic feed but, because there are shortages, some non-organic feed is currently allowed. For example, up to 10 per cent of a cow's diet, and a maximum of 20 per cent of chicken feed can be non-organic. Up to 60 per cent can come from sources that are in the process of converting to organic. There are plans to achieve 100 per cent organic feed by 2005.

In spite of all the evidence to the contrary, the UK government has taken action, mainly through the Food Standards Agency, to argue that there are no health benefits to eating organically produced foods. The following is an extract from another article in *Which?* magazine, in April 2002:[40]

The health benefits of eating fruit and vegetables are clear. The government wants us to eat at least five portions a day. To encourage this the Department of Health has introduced the National School Fruit Scheme, with the aim that, by 2004, all schoolchildren aged four to six will be receiving a piece of free fruit daily.

But fruit and vegetables tested still contain pesticide residues. Although most residues fall within legal safety levels, figures show 72 per cent of apples and 81 per cent of pears have residues. And, in December [2001] it was reported that 61 per cent of grapes and 63 per cent of kiwi fruit contained toxic chemicals. Exposure to pesticides may be linked to increasing cancer rates and other health problems – young children, in particular, may be more vulnerable.

The Food Standards Agency (FSA) has even established a working group to look at the 'cocktail effect' of multiple residues.

With these concerns, you'd expect the current and longstanding advice to wash and peel fruit as 'a sensible additional precaution when preparing fruit for small children' to be emphasised or improved. Instead, the FSA wants to ditch the advice because its 'misinterpretation' could imply that 'only organic fruit should be supplied to the National School Fruit Scheme' – according to a leaked memo.

However, the FSA told *Which?* that it was 'coincidental' that the advice was being reviewed prior to the launch of the school scheme and that it 'wasn't a trigger' for the review. It said that, since 1997, pesticide approval systems have been amended to take into account the variability of residue levels, and pesticide withdrawals have also taken place. It said that these changes could be sufficient grounds for the advice to be withdrawn.

It's important for us all to eat more fruit and vegetables, but this should not mean we are exposed to unnecessary health risks.

Which? thinks that the FSA approach isn't good enough and asks the government to be more transparent about its motives.

Based on known levels of pesticide residues in some fruit and vegetables, *Which?* magazine urges the continued adoption of precautionary washing and peeling – which also reinforces good hygiene – to remain in place.

HE WHO PAYS THE PIPER

So why is the UK Dairy Council being allowed to make claims that 'A natural fat [CLAs] found in milk, cheese, yoghurts and butter may soon prove to contain anti-cancer properties', when, as the *Sunday Times* article points out, 'the proportion of CLAs is only 1 in 120 parts of saturated fat; ergo, to come by a significant amount of CLAs, you'd have to eat artery-choking amounts of the fat stuff?[41]

In *Your Life in Your Hands* Jane warned about the consequences of the privatisation of science. Interestingly, the *Sunday Times* article makes the same point:

Of course, commercial science will look to where it's paid. 'CLA research was actually got going by the American meat and dairy industry', says Dr Campbell [Dr T. Colin

Campbell, professor emeritus at Cornell University, New York State, and a pioneer of dietary epidemiology], 'and it's very depressing when people start looking into little components of this and that. Let's face it, if dairy products contained all the good things that fruit and vegetables do, we'd be tired of hearing about them by now'.

PILLS AND POTIONS

What about the benefits of the osteoporosis epidemic to the vitamin and mineral manufacturers?

There is no doubt that they have been quick to jump on the high-calcium, high-magnesium, high-vitamin-D bandwagon. Many of the products have names suggesting protection against bone disease, and there are many websites devoted to promoting and marketing them. Quite simply, if you need to take these pills there is something wrong with your diet. The only exception is that vegans living in high latitudes should, in the winter, take extra vitamin D. The same may apply to people, such as some Muslim women, who keep their bodies almost entirely covered.

But let us look at another beneficiary of the osteoporosis epidemic. Let us look at the findings of Theta Report No. 940, October 1999. Theta Reports[42] is a division of PJB Publications, Ltd, publisher of *Scrip World Pharmaceutical News* and *Clinical World Medical Device & Diagnostic News*.

Theta Reports has provided high-quality comprehensive market research reports for business development, marketing, and research and development professionals since 1970. Focusing on pharmaceutical markets, biotech markets, medical device markets, and diagnostic markets, Theta's business reports identify market opportunities created by new and emerging technology. Our healthcare business reports define market size, project future growth, analyze products and market forces, and profile the key players to give you a competitive edge. We can also produce custom reports . . .

A study released in October 1999 by Theta Reports reveals that over 1.5 million hip, spine, and wrist fractures in the United States are due to osteoporosis. Further, more than 200 million people worldwide (80 per cent of these being female) are at risk for this condition.

Theta's report, *HRT/Osteoporosis Market* describes several new diagnostic and therapeutic technologies for this condition, which afflicts primarily older women. **The total market for osteoporosis treatments was worth $2.1 billion in 1998, and growing at an annual rate of close to 30 per cent per year** [our bold], despite the fact that only 20 per cent of those at risk for this condition have been diagnosed. Drug therapies (none of which have yet been approved for men) accounted for 95 per cent of this revenue. **The two major factors driving the growth of this market** [our bold] are: the aging of the population in general, and increasing awareness of women's health issues among both patients and physicians. Theta expects this market to continue to grow rapidly, as more individuals at potential risk for osteoporosis get evaluated. Further, several new therapies are being developed. This report reviews many of these, including: hormone replacement therapy (HRT), bisphosphonates and calcitonin.

Even the WHO definition is being used as a marketing tool for pharmaceuticals. The WHO definitions for Normal and Low Bone Mineral Density and Osteoporosis[43] (see page 4) were developed for epidemiologic studies but have been adopted as 'diagnostic criteria' in much the same way that arbitrarily selected cut-off points are used to define hypercholesterolemia (high blood cholesterol) and hypertension (high blood pressure). However, in our litigious society, bone mineral density more than 2 units below the mean is sometimes seen as the practical cut-off point for intervention. In fact, some drugs in the USA which were recently approved by the Food and Drug Administration for treatment of osteoporosis carry product labelling information indicating that a bone mineral density of −2 is appropriate for starting therapy.[44]

In the particular case of ERT/HRT, John Lee writes:[45]

Moreover, the pharmaceutical industry viewed the potential osteoporosis market as a magnificent opportunity to sell their patent medicine hormones. Doctors were treated to massive advertising campaigns via journal advertisements, promotional symposia disguised as 'continuing medical education' (i.e., CME, a requirement for physicians these days) with appropriate credits, personal visits by drug salesmen bringing boxes of free samples, and medical articles of studies spawned by generous grants from the industry, all touting the putative bone benefit of oestrogen and the protective effect (against endometrial cancer) of progestins. In the past few years, Prior et al. have provided reliable evidence that osteoporotic bone loss occurs in women with progesterone deficiency despite adequate oestrogen levels,[46] yet physicians continue to be taught that oestrogen is the single most potent factor in prevention of bone loss.[47] The strength of the oestrogen-fixed mindset represents a victory of advertising over science.

There are also videos, exercise books and even weighted vests (for weight-bearing exercise) – not to mention manufacture and use of DEXA and other diagnostic machines and methods and all the scientists being paid to do research (including unpleasant experiments on animals). Can it really be that the scourge of osteoporosis which is causing untold human misery in illness, deformity and loss of independence – not to mention the social and economic costs – is seen as a market opportunity by others?

But what about the medical professionals? Surely if one of the major factors in osteoporosis is to reduce animal protein in the diet they would be telling us to do this instead of (yes, really!) telling us to eat more dairy, including (and sometimes especially) cheese. So many of our friends, when we give them our advice, find it difficult to take it in because it conflicts so much with that of medical doctors, nurses and dieticians – although not that of scientists. According to one source in the USA:[48]

The dairy industry has a powerful hold on the nutrition industry in this country; it pays huge numbers of dieticians, doctors, and researchers to push dairy, spending more than $300 million annually, just at the national level, to retain a market for its products. **The dairy industry has infiltrated schools, bought off sports stars, celebrities, and politicians, pushing all the while an agenda based on profit, rather than public health** [our bold].

In a recent osteoporosis report in *The Practitioner*[49] there was no mention of animal protein as a potential risk factor.

Let us end this section with a quotation from one of the world's leading natural scientists of all time:

Great is the power of steady misrepresentation

Charles Darwin, 1872[50]

TEN GOLDEN GUIDELINES

How can we, as individuals, do anything to fight these powerful vested interests to improve our own bone health and cut the toll of osteoporosis on society as a whole? How can we give science victory over the pervasive influence of powerful interest groups? Below we give you ten golden guidelines to help in this fight.

1. Make good food ingredients your top priority when it comes to spending money. Keep as closely as you can to the Osteoporosis Plant Programme and wherever and whenever possible be prepared to pay extra for organically grown food produced as naturally as possible or grow your own. This sends the clearest possible message to government and the food industry. If you live in the UK try to buy food certified by the Soil Association from local sources as much as possible. The Internet is a very good way of finding local suppliers. If you buy organic food flown from distant countries, this increases pollution and there is no guarantee that the food is grown to standards such as those of the Soil Association.

2. Eat only those foods which human adults have evolved to eat. Most crucially leave out dairy produce which is designed for baby calves, goats or lambs, which can contain far too much calcium and growth factors such as IGF-1 and EPO which may cause excessive bone remodelling. Make sure you have adequate quantities of vegetables and fruit in your diet. Also refuse to eat food depleted of nutrients or otherwise altered by food processing, including food and drink which contain artificial chemical additives such as colouring and flavouring agents, preservatives and emulsifiers or food which has been chemically altered, for example fats which have been hydrogenated. Refuse to be bamboozled by marketing and advertising, look for the 'weasel words' and separate them in your mind from the underlying facts. Be suspicious – check labels and demand information.

3. Make eating good and nutritious meals based on wholesome nutritional ingredients your top priority when it comes to your time. The meals in Section 2 of this book can form part of a bone-protective lifestyle. Saving money to acquire material possessions to demonstrate a sophisticated lifestyle and saving time to further your career ambitions are probably two of the fundamental causes of osteoporosis (or breast cancer) in career women. A favourite novel is George Eliot's *Middlemarch*, and we should perhaps try to be more like Dorothea and less like Rosamund!

4. Try to keep alcohol within sensible limits. Do not binge, although social drinking in moderation, especially with meals, is fine. Avoid tobacco smoke, but if you can't quit nicotine, chew nicotine gum or use nicotine patches instead of smoking. Be concerned and take action to improve the environment for everybody. There are many chemicals being introduced that we can do nothing about as individuals. Collectively, we can reduce the impact of chemicals on the environment by reducing our use of materials such as perfumes and cosmetics, fluoridated tooth products, soft plastics, detergents, cleaning products and house and garden chemicals, and man-made fibres. Remember how in the past we were sold 'wonder' chemicals such as DDT and PCBs which have turned out to cause serious problems to the health of man, animals and the environment and which are still with us? What chemicals are we using today that scientists will have a similar view of in the future?

5. Take a little time to understand some basic science. Usually it is your money that scientists are spending directly or indirectly, and you need to understand what they are doing. Ensure that scientists contribute more to the public understanding of science by asking questions. If you do not understand the answer do not be embarrassed to repeat your question until you get a satisfactory answer. If scientists cannot explain their work properly it is their problem, not yours. Women, in particular, frequently throw up their hands at the very mention of science and say how unscientific they are – as if to admit knowing anything about science is unfeminine. It is essential that a well-informed body of opinion exists if science is to be directed for the benefit of humankind rather than lead to our downfall. It is vital that women, in particular, are involved in the direction of science for the good of society. Books that will 'fire you up' are *Silent Spring* by Rachel Carson, *Our Stolen Futures* by Colborn, Dumanski and Myers and *Planetary Overload* by A. J. McMichael. If you want to become more involved as lay members of the boards of scientific organisations, write in and offer your services, or you could consider joining the Consumer's Association which is run by professionals who have a balanced and honest approach to most issues concerning food and the environment. If there is a controversy about food or drink between the Consumer's Association and the Food Standards Agency, remember that it is the former that is actually funded by the consumer.

6. Learn to understand your basic anatomy and be aware of any marked changes in your weight, height or posture. Stand in front of a mirror and examine yourself regularly and keep records. This applies particularly to women after the menopause, but osteoporosis can strike men and women at any age. If you are on any of the long-term medications listed in Chapter 1, or have any of the medical conditions listed there, or have a family history of osteoporosis, ensure that you discuss these risk factors with your doctor and other health professionals. If you are over fifty, arrange a health check by a doctor or nurse once a year at a Well-Woman or Well-Man clinic, which most good general medical practices in the UK run.

7. Follow an exercise regime that you can keep to, one that is appropriate for your lifestyle, age and personality. Ideally spend as much time as possible out of doors – but do not expose skin, especially pale skin, to strong sunlight for too long.

8. If you are diagnosed with osteoporosis, use all the tools at your disposal to fight back. For your orthodox treatment ensure you are treated at a centre of excellence. Work with your doctor and be an involved and constructive participant in overcoming your illness, not a passive victim. Remember the many scientists and doctors quoted in this chapter who claim that osteoporosis can be treated and in some cases even reversed using the dietary and lifestyle factors described in this book.

9. Follow the diet and the lifestyle recommendations aimed at avoiding man-made chemicals as closely as possible. This includes minimising the use of non-prescription remedies available from pharmacies, such as antacids. If you are prescribed or recommended drugs by your doctor, ensure that you know precisely how they work and what the side effects are, especially if you need to take them over the long term. Take them only if you are satisfied with the explanation and convinced that there is no alternative. If your physician cannot explain how the drugs work and give examples of their successes and failures, be sceptical. Try to work with your health professionals to identify and eliminate the underlying cause of your illness, especially if this could involve some type of allergy or food intolerance.

10. Use methods such as meditation, hypnotherapy, visualisation and yoga to cope with any emotional distress and to develop the most positive approach possible. But do not rely on positive thinking alone. It is changing your body chemistry by changing your diet and lifestyle that is the crucial thing to do. Talk to your friends and family members and allow their help and support into your life, but if they find difficulty in coping, understand that they are distressed. Forgive them and allow them back into your life as soon as they feel able to return.

Knowledge is power. In this section of the book we have tried to empower both women and men to deal with osteoporsis, to take charge of the illness, ideally to prevent as many people as possible from contracting the disease. We hope very much that you can put this information to the best possible use in your life.

1 The Osteoporosis Plant Programme Cookbook

*The main purpose of this section of the book is to present more than a hundred recipes for delicious meals that are also good for bone health. The section includes principles of the cookbook and advice on a new shopping list aimed at restocking your cupboard and on essential equipment. The recipes are structured to help you balance the acidity and alkalinity of your diet. **All of the recipes are for four people unless otherwise stated.***

PRINCIPLES OF THE COOKBOOK

Many diets are difficult to keep to because the recipes are bland and boring and in some cases the regimes are harsh and extreme. With the Osteoporosis Plant Programme, in contrast, we have developed an exciting range of recipes based on the principles described in the previous section and inspired particularly by Asian cooking. The ready availability of Asian ingredients now makes it easy for everyone to adopt this delicious, healthy way of eating, based on an 'East meets West' style, which Gill, in particular, came to love and master while cooking for her family when she lived in Australia. Asian-style recipes often look complicated because they have a lot of ingredients, many of which are spices and herbs, but don't let this put you off. If you have a tray of all your spices to hand it is only about adding a few ingredients – it doesn't take a lot of time or make the dish complicated – it just improves flavour. Some healthy diets eliminate all spices, although many spices, such as saffron, contain antioxidants, and substances like circumin (in turmeric) have anti-cancer properties. Thai people have one of the lowest rates of bone fracture on record and Thai food is certainly spicy. The Ayurvedic medical system, which has been used for centuries in India, also uses many spices.

The style of cooking used here ensures that fresh, wholesome ingredients are cooked in the healthiest way possible and served while everything is still fresh. Also we recommend that you:

● **Never use a microwave cooker, because free radicals can be formed in the food**
● **Never use a pressure cooker, because vitamins and other important nutrients can be destroyed**

The style of cooking encourages social interaction. Women today do not want to be relegated to the kitchen away from families and friends. The recipes that follow are based on a modern style of living, kitchens are open plan and everyone is encouraged to join in, chat to the cook and have a drink – in moderation, of course. Once you have adapted to asking a partner or friend to chop this or that, or encouraged your children to add something to the pan, you will enjoy cooking in a more open sociable environment. You will relax because everyone has played a part in creating the meal, even if it is just by chatting to the cook.

CUSTOMISING THE RECIPES

All the recipes contain a full list of ingredients, but we recommend you use them only as a guide and add or subtract ingredients to develop the meals that you enjoy the most.

Remember:
● Any vegetable can be replaced with others. Use your favourite, what's in season or what is in the fridge. For example, change asparagus for beans and vice versa.
● Although the recipes are based on measured quantities, there are no hard and fast rules. Use what is left in a packet, or omit ingredients if you do not like their taste. You can do this without significantly changing the recipe.
● Herbs and spices are a matter of personal preference, so vary the quantities according to your likes and dislikes. If you like spicy food we think you will enjoy the recipes as presented, but

if you like milder food, simply cut down on the amount of spices, particularly chilli, and replace them with extra fresh herbs.

The chapter includes a comprehensive set of recipes. Also, many of your favourite meals may meet the principles of the programme or be adapted easily. Here are some simple changes to help you to make your usual meals healthier:

● **According to those great cooks Claudia Roden* and Marcella Hazan, 'it is quite possible to substitute olive oil for butter in almost any dish'.**
● **Soya 'milk' or 'cream' can be substituted for dairy milk or cream in most recipes.**
● **Solid vegetable oil or grapeseed oil can substitute for butter to make pastry or cakes.**
● **Balance the acid and alkaline components of your meals. For example, eat rice and pasta mainly with vegetables rather than meat, fish or eggs, or have a large bowl of vegetable soup before a meat dish.**
● **Use your local farm shop or organic food supplier. Not only will you be buying healthier food, but you will be helping local industry, reducing the transport-related output of greenhouse gases, and doing your bit for the environment, as well as for yourself.**

In order to help you to begin, the recipes have been organised into suggestions for breakfasts, snacks and lunches or meals on the run and main meals. But most of the meals taste just as good at other times of the day. For example, the soups described in the 'Meals on the Run' section could be a full meal, a starter for dinner, or even a different breakfast.

The recipes previously published in *The Plant Programme* are just as good for the prevention and treatment of osteoporosis. They can be used to complement those in this book, although in some of them you might wish to replace rice or cereal with potato to reduce the acid-forming component of the meal. The

---

*Roden, Claudia, 1968. *A New Book of Middle Eastern Food.* Penguin Books, 11.

Osteoporosis Plant Programme also recommends the use of chicken and fish bones in making stocks for soups.

ESSENTIAL EQUIPMENT

We are assuming you have the usual range of cooking utensils, pots and pans, knives etc. However, here are some things you may not have, that will help make the recipes easier to prepare:

● FOOD PROCESSOR – there are many to choose from, the two most important functions are chopping and puréeing
● GARLIC PRESS
● HAND-HELD BLENDER AND FOOD-PROCESSOR ATTACHMENT – we find this the most useful piece of equipment in the kitchen. It is great for chopping small quantities of herbs, nuts, garlic or ginger, and for blending soups, making pastes, etc.
● ICE-CREAM MAKER (optional) – most of the sorbets and ice 'creams' in this book have been made with a hand-turned ice-cream maker with a metal freezer bowl, which is kept in the freezer
● JUICE EXTRACTOR
● METRIC MEASURING CUPS AND SPOONS
● MICROPLANE GRATER – brilliant for grating ginger and lemon peel
● MINCER (optional) – if you want to mince your own ingredients this is a very useful piece of equipment. Ours have a citrus squeezer and different sized graters as attachments and we use them regularly
● PEPPER AND SALT MILLS
● SIEVES – to rinse rice, drain pasta, strain soups, wash fruit, etc.
● SALAD SHAKER – to dry salad vegetables easily, and prevent watering down the dressing
● CHARGRILL PAN – a ridged, flat frying pan that is a quick and easy alternative to a barbecue. Perfect for grilling prawns or squid and vegetables. Large electric ones are now available
● SAUTÉ PAN WITH LID
● STEAMER WITH LID
● NON-STICK WOK WITH LID

THE RESTOCKED CUPBOARD

This section gives an indicative shopping list, which includes most of the ingredients used in the recipes. You do not need to have everything, but it is particularly helpful to have the spices and herbs to hand.

When shopping, ensure that you read all labels carefully and avoid anything that contains milk solids, lactose, whey, casein, milk, yoghurt, cheese or other dairy ingredients. One brand of food may be dairy free, while another brand of the same food will contain dairy. We have found that 'Naan', a traditional Indian bread contains yoghurt when found in the supermarkets, while if you buy it from an Indian supermarket, it doesn't. Also, some Japanese powdered dashi (soup stock) available in Asian shops in Britain can contain lactose. The dairy additives are cheap fillers and would not be found in traditional Asian food.

THE ALKALINE-ACID HIERARCHY

We present our shopping list in order of increasing acid-generating potential: foods at the top of the list are highly alkaline and you can have plenty of them, while those at the bottom are the most acid and you should eat them only in the balance described on page 100 to prevent or treat osteoporosis:

1 Herbs and spices
2 Fruit and vegetables
3 Beverages
4 Fats and oils: non-dairy 'milk', 'cream', 'yoghurt' and spreads
5 Sugars
6 Legumes, nuts, seeds and grains
7 Meat, fish, shellfish, poultry and eggs

HERBS AND SPICES
FRESH
● Basil
● Bay leaves
● Chillies, red and green
● Chives
● Coriander
● Curry leaves

- Garlic
- Ginger
- Lemon grass
- Lime leaves
- Mint
- Parsley
- Rosemary
- Sage
- Thai basil
- Thyme

Fresh herbs and spices, including garlic, ginger, lime leaves, lemon grass, parsley and bay leaves, can be frozen. Wrap them in foil and keep in the freezer until needed. They are most easily chopped or sliced while still frozen.

DRY

- Bay leaves
- Black pepper
- Cardamom
- Cayenne or chilli powder
- Cinnamon, sticks and ground
- Cloves
- Coriander powder
- Cumin powder
- Garam masala
- Mustard seeds
- Nutmeg
- Paprika
- Saffron
- Sea salt
- Tamarind
- Turmeric

BOTTLED OR CANNED

- Curry paste
- Chilli sambal (minced chilli)
- Thai sweet chilli sauce

FRUIT

ANY FRESH FRUIT, INCLUDING:

- Apples
- Bananas
- Berries
- Figs
- Grapefruit
- Grapes
- Kiwi fruit
- Mandarins (clementines, tangerines)
- Mango
- Melon (cantaloupe, galia)
- Nectarines
- Oranges
- Papaya
- Passion fruit
- Peaches
- Pears
- Pineapple
- Plums
- Pomegranate
- Pomelo
- Watermelon

ANY FROZEN FRUIT without added sugar
FRESHLY SQUEEZED FRUIT JUICES
DRIED FRUIT – buy the unsulphured varieties
- Apricots
- Currants
- Dates
- Figs
- Prunes
- Raisins

VEGETABLES
ANY FRESH VEGETABLE INCLUDING:
- Aubergine
- Avocado
- Bean sprouts
- Beetroot
- Bok choy (pak choi)
- Broccoli
- Cabbage
- Carrots
- Cauliflower
- Celery
- Celeriac
- Chicory
- Choi sum
- Corn on the cob, baby corn
- Cucumber
- Fennel
- Green beans
- Leeks
- Lettuce, all types
- Mushrooms
- Mustard greens

- Onions, red and brown
- Parsnips
- Peppers, red, green, orange and yellow
- Potatoes
- Pumpkin
- Rocket
- Snap peas
- Snow peas
- Spinach
- Sweet potato
- Tomatoes, vine-ripened varieties
- Watercress
- Zucchini
FROZEN
- Corn
- Peas
BOTTLED OR CANNED
- Artichokes in olive oil
- Bamboo shoots
- Water chestnuts
DRIED
- Chinese mushrooms
- Seaweed (kombu, wakame, nori)
- Shiitake mushrooms
- Sun-dried or sun-blush tomatoes

BEVERAGES
- Herb teas
- Green tea
- Pure cocoa
- Filtered water and good-quality mineral waters in glass bottles
- Beer

- Cider
- Red and white wine

OILS
- Olive oil
- Sesame oil
- Soya spread
- Sunflower spread
- Grapeseed oil
- Walnut oil
- Coconut milk
- Coconut cream
- Peanut butter
- Rice, oat or pea milk
- Soya milk, cream and yoghurt
- Soya spread

SUGARS
- Raw organic honey and maple syrup
- Organic jams and marmalades (best made with fruit concentrate rather than sugar)
- Organic unrefined sugar or molasses
- Dark chocolate (dairy free)

LEGUMES
- Beans (cannellini, kidney, etc.)
- Bean curd (tofu)
- Chickpeas
- Lentils
- Miso
- Split peas
- Tempeh

NUTS
- Almonds
- Coconut
- Hazelnuts
- Pine nuts
- Walnuts

SEEDS
- Pumpkin seeds
- Sesame seeds
- Sunflower seeds

GRAINS
- Barley
- Couscous
- Crispbreads
- Egg pasta and noodles
- Naan
- Oats
- Pastry
- Pitta bread
- Polenta
- Rice (arborio, basmati, sushi, wild)
- Rice noodles
- Spring roll wrappers
- Tortillas
- Wholemeal and rye breads
- Wholemeal and strong white flour

SAUCES AND SEASONINGS
- Balsamic vinegar
- Capers
- Chinese cooking wine
- Cider vinegar
- Fish sauce

- Furikake Japanese seasoning
- Instant miso soup powder
- Light soya sauce
- Mirin
- Organic stock cubes (vegetable and chicken)
- Organic tomato ketchup
- Organic tomato paste
- Shoyu sauce
- Tamari sauce
- Teriyaki sauce
- Wasabi paste or powder
- Wine vinegar (red and white)

FISH AND SEAFOOD

All fish and seafood including:
- Cod
- Crab
- Wild (not farmed) salmon
- Haddock
- Ocean trout
- Prawns
- Scallops
- Sea bass
- Sole
- Squid
- Tuna

MEAT AND POULTRY (ORGANIC WHEREVER POSSIBLE)

- Beef
- Chicken
- Duck
- Eggs
- Lamb
- Pork
- Rabbit
- Venison

WEIGHTS AND MEASURES

Conversions used for the
recipes in this book are: 1 tbsp = 15 ml
¼ cup = 60 ml   1 oz = 30 g
½ cup = 125 ml   4 oz = 125 g
1 cup = 250 ml   8 oz = 250 g
1 tsp = 5 ml   1 lb = 500 g

APPROXIMATE OVEN TEMPERATURES

	°C	°F	Mark
Very cool or very slow	135°C	275°F	1
Cool or slow	150°C	300°F	2–3
Moderate	180°C	350°F	4–5
Hot	200°C	400°F	6–7
Very hot	220°C	425°F	8

DAILY AND WEEKLY MENU PLANNER

The simple guidelines are:
- Start the day with fresh fruit and vegetable juice.
- About 75 per cent of daily intake to be fruit and vegetables, including cereals, nuts and pulses (such as peas and beans).
- Minimise acid tides in the body by ensuring that meals are pH balanced. For example do not have a meal comprising only meat and pasta, especially with cheese – all of which are acid-generating foods.

	Breakfast	Lunch	Dinner
Monday	Apricot compote. Blueberry muffins	Avocado and tomato bruschetta	Chicken laksa
Tuesday	Pear and watermelon juice. Grilled mushrooms on toast	Chicken salad	Sautéed cauliflower with tomato and capers
Wednesday	Apple and kiwifruit juice. Muesli with soya milk and mixed berries	Crispy green salad, wholemeal roll	Chicken teriyaki Garlic spinach. Baked sweet potato
Thursday	Slice of melon or papaya. Grilled tomatoes on toasted wholemeal bread	Crab and cucumber salad	Zucchini and pea curry. Potato and aubergine curry
Friday	Strawberry, melon and kiwifruit salad. Toast and honey	Asian noodle and watercress salad	Fish stew
Saturday	Coconut pancakes with grilled banana	Spicy aubergine with baked potato	Pork satay. Sesame green beans
Sunday	Carrot, celery and tomato juice. Hash browns with poached egg and spinach	Roast lamb loin with grilled vegetables	Chilled avocado soup

2 Recipes

- *No dairy – especially cheese*
- *Plenty of fresh fruit and vegetables*
- *Only 20 per cent of food intake to be protein if you have osteoporosis*
- *Less than 40 per cent of food intake to be protein for osteoporosis prevention*

Do not become so extreme in your eating habits that you become protein deficient.

GOOD BEGINNINGS

All fruit and vegetables are alkaline and therefore fresh fruit and vegetable juice, and/ or a fresh fruit salad are a good way to start the day. Even those who don't like vegetables generally enjoy them in the combinations suggested below.

FRUIT AND VEGETABLE JUICE SUGGESTIONS:
- Apple, carrot and celery juice
- Apple, celery and mandarin juice
- Cucumber, green pepper and pear juice
- Grapefruit and celery juice
- Orange, apple, and strawberry juice
- Papaya, banana and apple juice
- Pear and strawberry juice
- Tomato, carrot and celery juice

APRICOT COMPOTE
PREPARATION TIME: 1 minute
COOKING TIME: 10–15 minutes

HERBS AND SPICES
1/4 tsp ground cinnamon

ALKALINE
200 g dried apricots

NEARLY NEUTRAL
2 tbsp sugar
$\frac{1}{2}$ cup water
Soya yoghurt

Put the apricots in a pan, sprinkle over the sugar and cinnamon, add the water, bring to the boil and simmer for about 10–15 minutes. Serve with soya yoghurt.

AVOCADO AND TOMATO BRUSCHETTA
PREPARATION TIME: 5 minutes
COOKING TIME: 2–3 minutes

HERBS AND SPICES
1–2 garlic cloves, peeled
$\frac{1}{4}$ cup chopped fresh basil

ALKALINE
2 avocados, peeled and stoned
2–3 vine-ripened tomatoes, sliced
1 tsp lemon juice

NEARLY NEUTRAL
2 tsp olive oil

ACID
4 slices Italian bread, toasted

Rub the garlic clove over the toast. Mash the avocado, sprinkle it with the lemon juice and spread it on the toast. Toss the tomato slices in the olive oil, place them on the avocado and serve sprinkled with chopped basil.

BANANA MILK SHAKE (serves 1)
PREPARATION TIME: 1 minute

HERBS AND SPICES
Freshly grated nutmeg

ALKALINE
1 banana, peeled and sliced

NEARLY NEUTRAL
1 cup soya milk
1 tsp honey (optional)

Blend the banana, soya milk and honey with a hand-held blender
or using a food processor. Serve sprinkled with grated nutmeg.

VARIATIONS *Use strawberries, mango, papaya, or any other soft
fruit or any combination of fruits.*

BANANA BREAD
PREPARATION TIME: 10 minutes
COOKING TIME: 55–60 minutes

HERBS AND SPICES
½ tsp ground cinnamon

ALKALINE
3 ripe bananas, mashed

NEARLY NEUTRAL
1 cup soya milk
½ cup raw brown cane sugar
2 tbsp sunflower oil

ACID
2 eggs
2 cups self-raising flour
1 tsp baking powder

Preheat the oven to 170°C. Lightly beat the eggs then add the
bananas, soya milk, sugar and oil and mix together. Sift the
flour, baking powder, and cinnamon into a bowl and roughly
fold in the egg mixture. Pour the mixture into a lightly oiled

loaf tin. Bake for 55–60 minutes or until a skewer inserted in the middle comes out clean.

BERRY SMOOTHIE (serves 1–2)
PREPARATION TIME: 1–2 minutes

ALKALINE
1 cup fresh orange or apple juice
1 cup fresh or frozen berries
1 large banana

NEARLY NEUTRAL
1 tsp honey (optional)

Blend all the ingredients together using a hand-held blender or food processor.

VARIATIONS *Replace berries with any other fruit.*

FRUIT MUFFINS
This recipe was given to us by Chris Williams.
PREPARATION TIME: 5 minutes
COOKING TIME: 20–25 minutes

ALKALINE
1 cup blueberries or chopped apple

NEARLY NEUTRAL
$3/4$–1 cup soya milk or fresh fruit juice
$1/3$ cup grapeseed oil
$1/2$ cup sugar

ACID
1 large egg
2 cups wholemeal flour
1 tbsp baking powder

Preheat the oven to 200°C. Lightly grease a muffin tin or line it with muffin cups. Sieve together the flour, sugar and baking powder. Lightly whisk together the soya milk, egg and oil, then gently fold in the flour ingredients (you don't need to mix them too well). Add the blueberries or apple and again fold gently into the mixture. Divide the mixture between the muffin cups, filling them about ⅔ full. Bake for about 20–25 minutes or until a toothpick inserted into the middle comes out clean. Allow to cool for 1 minute before removing from the pan.

TIP 25 per cent of flour can be replaced with oatmeal in most recipes to improve your magnesium intake.

GRILLED TOMATOES WITH PESTO ON TOAST
PREPARATION TIME: 1 minute
COOKING TIME: 3–4 minutes

HERBS AND SPICES
Chopped fresh basil or oregano (optional)

ALKALINE
1–2 tomatoes per person

NEARLY NEUTRAL
Pesto*

ACID
4 slices wholemeal toast

Cut the tomatoes in half and grill. Toast the bread, spread with pesto and top with the grilled tomatoes. Serve garnished with basil or oregano.

*PESTO
PREPARATION TIME: 5 minutes

HERBS AND SPICES
2 cups loosely packed fresh basil leaves

2–3 cloves garlic, peeled

NEARLY NEUTRAL
$\frac{1}{4}$–$\frac{1}{2}$ cup olive oil

ACID
$\frac{1}{2}$ cup pine nuts

Blend all the ingredients together in a food processor to form a thick paste.

NOTE Pesto will keep in the fridge for up to a week.

HOME-MADE TOASTED MUESLI
This recipe was given to us by Chris Williams. Oats are excellent sources of calcium, magnesium and other trace nutrients, but are acid forming. This muesli is therefore balanced with dried fruit and you can increase the alkalinity further by serving with fresh fruit such as sliced banana.
PREPARATION TIME: 10 minutes
COOKING TIME: 45 minutes

ALKALINE
1 cup dried apricots cut into slivers
200 g raisins
100 g grated coconut

NEARLY NEUTRAL
220 ml honey
200 ml grapeseed oil

ACID
400 g rolled oats
100 g almond slivers

Preheat the oven to 180°C. Mix together all the ingredients except the honey and grapeseed oil in a large oven-proof dish. Mix together the honey and grapeseed oil and warm them through, then mix them with the other ingredients. Bake in the oven until the oats are a light brown colour, stirring the mixture about every 15 minutes to avoid the bottom layer burning. Turn off the oven but leave the muesli in to cool. Serve with soya milk or soya yoghurt.

Store in a dry cool place in an airtight container for up to a month.

HOME-MADE MUESLI
Cereals are acid forming, but the addition of fresh fruit, raisins and spices helps to balance this dish.
PREPARATION TIME: 10 minutes
COOKING TIME: 1–2 minutes

HERBS AND SPICES
1 tsp ground cinnamon
¼ tsp ground nutmeg

ALKALINE
2 small Granny Smith apples, grated
1 tsp lemon juice
1½ cups fresh apple or orange juice
1 cup raisins
1 punnet blueberries or other berries in season

NEARLY NEUTRAL
1 cup soya yoghurt or soya milk
2 tsp honey (optional) or to taste
¼ cup sesame seeds
¼ cup sunflower seeds

ACID
2 cups rolled oats
¼ cup slivered almonds

Toast the almonds, sesame and sunflower seeds in the oven or in a pan for a few minutes. Sprinkle the grated apple with lemon juice. Mix together all the ingredients except the blueberries. Cover and refrigerate overnight (this is actually quite delicious after only about 10 minutes soaking). Serve with extra soya yoghurt or soya milk and fresh blueberries.

MUSHROOMS WITH OLIVE PASTE (TAPENADE) ON TOAST

PREPARATION TIME: 5 minutes
COOKING TIME: 5 minutes

HERBS AND SPICES
Chopped fresh parsley to garnish
Pepper to taste

ALKALINE
4–8 field mushrooms, peeled
2 tbsp olive paste*

NEARLY NEUTRAL
1–2 tsp olive oil

ACID
4 slices wholemeal bread

Sprinkle a little olive oil over the top of the mushrooms and then grill or sauté until cooked. Toast the bread, spread with the olive paste and top with the cooked mushrooms. Serve garnished with a little chopped parsley and season to taste.

*OLIVE PASTE

PREPARATION TIME: 10–15 minutes depending on whether or not you have to stone the olives.

HERBS AND SPICES
2–3 cloves garlic, peeled
²/₃ cup fresh wide-leaved parsley,
2 tbsp fresh rosemary leaves (stem removed)
2 tbsp fresh thyme leaves (stem removed)
1 tsp black pepper

ALKALINE
2 cups olives, stoned (Kalamata olives have the best flavour)
1 tbsp capers

NEARLY NEUTRAL
3 tbsp olive oil

Purée all the ingredients to a coarse paste in a food processor.

NOTE *Store any left-over olive paste in the fridge – it will keep for up to a week.*

POACHED EGGS WITH HASH BROWN POTATOES

Potatoes help to balance out the acidity of the eggs, but to increase the alkalinity of the meal, serve with grilled tomatoes or mushrooms.
PREPARATION TIME: 10 minutes
COOKING TIME: 25–30 minutes (if using uncooked potatoes)

HERBS AND SPICES
4–5 garlic cloves, crushed
2 tsp chopped fresh Italian or wide-leaved parsley
1 tsp dried thyme
Black pepper

ALKALINE
500 g potatoes,
4–5 spring onions, finely chopped

NEARLY NEUTRAL
3–4 tbsp olive oil

ACID
4 eggs

Parboil or steam the potatoes, cool, peel and grate coarsely (or use left-over potatoes). Heat the olive oil and sauté the garlic and spring onions for a minute, then remove them from the pan and add them to the potatoes with the parsley and thyme and stir gently to mix together well. Divide the potato mixture into balls and flatten slightly. Add the potato balls in batches to the pan and fry until they start to turn brown (add a little more oil if necessary), then turn the potato over and cook the other side. Meanwhile, half fill a frying pan with water and when gently simmering, break the eggs into individual poaching rings and cook for about 3 minutes or until done to your liking. Drain the eggs and serve on top of the hash brown potatoes.

POACHED PEACHES WITH PORRIDGE
PREPARATION TIME: 5 minutes
COOKING TIME: 15–20 minutes

ALKALINE
4–5 small peaches, stoned and cut into quarters
1 tbsp lemon juice

NEARLY NEUTRAL
$\frac{1}{4}$ cup raw cane sugar
Soya milk or soya yoghurt

ACID
Porridge oats

Prepare the porridge oats following the instructions on the packet. Put the peaches in a saucepan with the sugar and lemon juice and 2 tablespoons water and simmer gently for about 10 minutes or until the peaches are soft. Serve the porridge with the peaches and soya milk, soya yoghurt or, if you prefer, soya cream.

SCRAMBLED EGGS WITH GARLIC AND SPRING ONIONS
Eggs are acid forming, and although the garlic and spring onions help to balance the meal, serving them with grilled tomatoes,

mushrooms or hash brown potatoes rather than toast improves
the overall balance of the meal.
PREPARATION TIME: 5 minutes
COOKING TIME: 4–5 minutes

HERBS AND SPICES
3–4 garlic cloves, minced
1 green chilli (optional)
Pepper to taste
Chopped fresh coriander or parsley for garnish

ALKALINE
8 spring onions, finely sliced

NEARLY NEUTRAL
1 tbsp olive oil
1 tbsp soya milk
1 tbsp water

ACID
6 eggs

Lightly beat together the eggs, soya milk and water and season
to taste. Heat the oil and stir-fry the spring onions, garlic and
chilli for 1–2 minutes. Add the egg mixture and stir gently over
a medium heat until cooked to your liking. Serve garnished
with chopped coriander or parsley.

VARIATION *Replace the spring onions with finely chopped leek.*

STRAWBERRY, MELON, KIWIFRUIT AND SOYA YOGHURT SALAD
PREPARATION TIME: 5–6 minutes

ALKALINE
4 kiwifruit, peeled and sliced
300 g strawberries, sliced
½ Galia melon cut into cubes

NEARLY NEUTRAL
Soya yoghurt

Mix together the strawberries, melon and kiwifruit and sprinkle with lemon juice. Serve with soya yoghurt.

MEALS ON THE RUN

SOUPS

BASIC CHICKEN STOCK

Making your own stock is easy but time consuming, but once prepared it can be kept in the freezer. Home-made stock is an excellent natural source of calcium and other trace nutrients.
PREPARATION TIME: 5 minutes
COOKING TIME: 3 hours

HERBS AND SPICES
2–3 bay leaves
1 sprig fresh thyme
6 whole black peppercorns
3 stalks fresh parsley

ALKALINE
1 carrot, sliced
1 stick celery, sliced
1 onion, sliced
1 leek, sliced

ACID
1–2 chicken carcasses

Place all the chicken bones in a pan, cover with water, bring to a slow simmer, and skim any scum from the surface. Add all the other ingredients and continue to simmer gently for about 3 hours, topping up with water as necessary. Strain the stock and allow to cool. Remove any fat from the surface.

This stock will keep in the fridge for 2–3 days or it can be frozen.

BEAN CURD AND MUSHROOM SOUP

PREPARATION TIME: 5 minutes
COOKING TIME: 10 minutes

HERBS AND SPICES
4–5 garlic cloves, crushed
1 tbsp fresh ginger, grated
1 tsp chilli sambal or 1 red chilli, finely chopped
2 tbsp chopped fresh coriander

ALKALINE
4–5 spring onions, finely sliced
150 g fresh shiitake or chestnut mushrooms, sliced
1 bunch mustard greens or choi sum cut into 2 or 3 pieces

NEARLY NEUTRAL
2 tbsp groundnut oil
2 tbsp sesame oil
1 tbsp mirin
1 l chicken stock

ACID
250 g fresh bean curd, cut into thin slices
1 tbsp Chinese vinegar

Heat the groundnut oil and pan fry the bean curd for 2–3 minutes, then remove from pan and keep warm. In a separate saucepan, heat the sesame oil and sauté the garlic, ginger and chilli for one minute. Add the mushrooms and continue to sauté for another 2 minutes. Add the chicken stock, mirin and Chinese vinegar and bring to a gentle simmer. Add the mustard greens stalks and simmer for a further 2–3 minutes. Add the mustard green leaves and spring onions and continue to simmer until the leaves are just wilted (1–2 minutes). Put the bean curd slices in serving bowls, serve over the soup and vegetables and garnish with fresh coriander.

BEAN CURD AND SPINACH SOUP
PREPARATION TIME: 2 minutes
COOKING TIME: 5 minutes

HERBS AND SPICES
½ cup fresh coriander leaves, coarsely chopped

ALKALINE
100 g baby spinach leaves
2 spring onions, sliced diagonally

NEARLY NEUTRAL
1 l chicken stock
1 tbsp light soya sauce

ACID
120 g soft bean curd, drained

Cut the bean curd into small slices, about 5 mm thick. Bring the
stock to a gentle simmer, then add the bean curd and soya sauce
and cook for 2–3 minutes. Skim any scum from the surface.
Divide the spinach and spring onions among 4 serving bowls
and pour over the soup. Serve garnished with coriander leaves.

BROCCOLI AND LEMON GRASS SOUP
PREPARATION TIME: 10 minutes
COOKING TIME: 20 minutes

HERBS AND SPICES
3–4 garlic cloves, chopped
1 green chilli, sliced
1 stalk lemon grass, cut into 2½ cm lengths
2–3 lime leaves
Ground black pepper
Chopped fresh parsley or coriander

ALKALINE
1 onion, chopped

500 g broccoli, coarsely chopped and stems peeled
2 tbsp lemon juice

NEARLY NEUTRAL
3 tbsp olive oil
1½ l vegetable or chicken stock

Heat the olive oil and sauté the onion for 3–4 minutes. Add the garlic, chilli, lemon grass, lime leaves and broccoli stems and continue to sauté for 2 minutes. Add the stock and simmer for about 10 minutes. Add the broccoli florets and continue to cook for another 3–4 minutes. Remove the lime leaves and lemon grass and purée the soup. Add the lemon juice and serve garnished with chopped parsley or coriander and black pepper to taste.

BROCCOLI AND POTATO SOUP
PREPARATION TIME: 10 minutes
COOKING TIME: 35–40 minutes

HERBS AND SPICES
3–4 garlic cloves, chopped
Black pepper
Fresh basil leaves, coarsely chopped

ALKALINE
1 large onion, peeled and chopped
500 g potatoes, cleaned and diced
400 g broccoli, cut into small florets, and the stalks peeled and chopped

NEARLY NEUTRAL
4 tbsp olive oil
1¼ l stock

Sauté the onion in the olive oil for about 3–4 minutes, add the garlic and continue to sauté for another minute. Add the potatoes and broccoli stalks, stir and sauté for another 1–2 minutes. Add the stock, season to taste with black pepper, bring to a slow simmer, cover and simmer for about 20 minutes until the potatoes are soft and beginning to break up. Add the broccoli florets and simmer for another 3–4 minutes. Stir in the basil leaves and serve.

VARIATION Use 1 tbsp pesto instead of the basil leaves.

CARROT AND ZUCCHINI SOUP
PREPARATION TIME: 5 minutes
COOKING TIME: 20–25 minutes

HERBS AND SPICES
4–5 cloves garlic, chopped
1 tsp cumin powder
1 tsp paprika
Chopped fresh parsley for garnish

ALKALINE
2 medium brown onions, chopped
3–4 medium carrots, cleaned and sliced
2–3 medium zucchini, washed and sliced

NEARLY NEUTRAL
3 tbsp olive oil
1½ l vegetable or chicken stock

Heat the olive oil and sauté the onions for 3–4 minutes, add the garlic, cumin and paprika and continue to sauté for another minute. Add the carrots and zucchini and stir to ensure they are well coated in the oil and spices and continue to sauté for another 2–3 minutes. Add the stock, and simmer gently for about 15 minutes until the vegetables are soft. Serve with an extra sprinkle of cumin powder and parsley.

CHILLED AVOCADO SOUP
PREPARATION TIME: 5 minutes plus chilling time

HERBS AND SPICES
3–4 cloves garlic, crushed
½ tsp ground cumin
½ tsp ground coriander
1 green chilli
2 tbsp chopped fresh chives
Black pepper

ALKALINE
2 large ripe avocados, peeled and stoned
¼ cup lemon juice

NEARLY NEUTRAL
1 l chicken stock

Process all the ingredients, except the chives and the black pepper in a food processor until they form a smooth paste. Serve chilled, garnished with chives or other fresh herbs and freshly ground black pepper to taste.

CHILLED CUCUMBER SOUP
PREPARATION TIME: 5 minutes plus chilling time
COOKING TIME: 12–15 minutes

HERBS AND SPICES
4–5 garlic cloves, sliced
Black pepper to taste
½ cup chopped fresh chives

ALKALINE
1 small leek, washed and coarsely chopped
2 cucumbers, washed and coarsely chopped
Zest from 1 lemon
1 tbsp lemon juice

NEARLY NEUTRAL
2 tbsp olive oil
1 l chicken or vegetable stock

1 cup soya yoghurt

Sauté the leek in the olive oil for 2–3 minutes, add the garlic and continue to sauté for another minute. Add the cucumber and stir until it is coated in the oil, and sauté for another 3–4 minutes. Add the stock and simmer for 4–5 minutes. Purée the soup, stir in the yoghurt, lemon zest, and lemon juice, season to taste and refrigerate. Serve chilled garnished with the chives.

CHILLED LETTUCE AND MINTED PEA SOUP
PREPARATION TIME: 5 minutes plus chilling time
COOKING TIME: 15–20 minutes

HERBS AND SPICES
3–4 cloves garlic, crushed
½ long green chilli (optional) chopped
2 tbsp wide-leaved parsley, chopped
2 tbsp mint leaves, chopped
Black pepper to taste
2 tbsp chived, chopped

ALKALINE
1 onion, chopped
1 small romaine lettuce, roughly chopped

NEARLY NEUTRAL
2 tbsp olive oil
1 l chicken stock
4 tsp soya cream or soya yoghurt (optional)

ACID
200 g fresh or frozen peas

Heat the olive oil and sauté the onion for 3–4 minutes until soft. Add the garlic and chilli and continue to sauté for another minute. Add the lettuce and stir to coat in the oil and sauté for another minute. Add the peas and stock and simmer for about 10 minutes until the peas are cooked. Add the parsley and mint and continue to simmer for another minute, then purée and season to taste. Serve chilled, garnished with chopped chives and a swirl of soya cream or soya yoghurt.

CRAB AND ASPARAGUS SOUP
PREPARATION TIME: 2–3 minutes
COOKING TIME: 6–8 minutes

HERBS AND SPICES
1 tsp minced chilli or 1 red chilli finely chopped
$\frac{1}{2}$ tsp coarse black pepper
Chopped fresh coriander

ALKALINE
6–8 spring onions, finely sliced

NEARLY NEUTRAL
1 l chicken stock
16–20 stalks of asparagus, each cut into 4 slices
2 tsp fish sauce
1 tsp sesame oil

ACID
170 g tin of white crabmeat, drained and shredded
3 egg whites
Soya sauce or Chinese brown vinegar

Bring the stock to a gentle simmer, add the chilli and asparagus stalks and simmer for 3–4 minutes. Add the fish sauce, black pepper, asparagus tips, spring onions and crab meat and simmer for another 2 minutes. Lightly whisk the egg whites with the sesame oil. Turn off the heat under the soup and slowly stir in the egg whites. Serve immediately, garnished with chopped fresh coriander and soya sauce or Chinese brown vinegar to taste.

CRAB AND CORN SOUP
PREPARATION TIME: 5 minutes
COOKING TIME: 15 minutes

HERBS AND SPICES
1 tbsp fresh ginger, grated
½ cup chopped fresh coriander

ALKALINE
4 spring onions, finely sliced

NEARLY NEUTRAL
2 tbsp olive oil
1 l chicken stock
1 tbsp mirin
2 tsp sesame oil

ACID
2 cups fresh or frozen corn kernels, coarsely chopped in the food
    processor
1 can white crab meat, rinsed, drained and flaked
2 tbsp light soya sauce
1 tsp cornflour
1 egg
2 tsp Chinese brown vinegar

Heat the olive oil and stir-fry the ginger and spring onions for
about a minute. Add the chicken stock, corn, mirin and soya
sauce and simmer for 2–3 minutes. Add the crab and continue
to simmer for another 2 minutes. Mix the cornflour with a
little water to make a thin paste and pour this into the soup
and simmer for 2 minutes. Lightly beat the egg with the
sesame oil. Remove the soup from the heat, add the vinegar
and pour in the beaten egg slowly, stirring gently. Serve
immediately, garnished with freshly chopped coriander.

VARIATION *Use 2 poached chicken breasts, shredded, instead of
the crab, and add along with the stock.*

CURRIED CAULIFLOWER AND ZUCCHINI SOUP
PREPARATION TIME: 10 minutes
COOKING TIME: 20 minutes

HERBS AND SPICES
4–5 cloves garlic, chopped
1 tsp coriander powder
2 tsp cumin powder
1 tsp cayenne pepper
1 tsp garam masala
½ tsp turmeric
6–8 curry leaves (optional)
Pepper to taste
Chopped fresh coriander

ALKALINE
1 onion, chopped
1 small cauliflower, divided into florets
2 small zucchini, washed and sliced

NEARLY NEUTRAL
2 tbsp olive oil
1¼ l chicken stock, warm

Sauté the onion in the olive oil for 3–4 minutes, add the garlic
and all the spices except the fresh coriander, stir and continue
to sauté for 1–2 minutes. Add the cauliflower and zucchini and
stir until they are well coated with the spices and sauté for
another 1–2 minutes. Add the warm stock and simmer for
about 15 minutes or until the cauliflower is cooked. Purée,
adding a little more water if the soup is too thick, and reheat.
Season to taste and serve garnished with the coriander

VARIATION Use 1 tablespoon curry paste instead of the spices.

CURRIED PARSNIP SOUP
PREPARATION TIME: 10 minutes
COOKING TIME: 25–30 minutes

HERBS AND SPICES
4–5 garlic cloves, chopped
1 tbsp cumin powder
1 tbsp coriander powder

1 tsp cayenne pepper
½ tsp turmeric powder
Black pepper
Chopped fresh coriander

ALKALINE
1 onion, chopped
2 large parsnips, peeled and chopped

NEARLY NEUTRAL
2 tbsp olive oil
1¼ l chicken stock

Sauté the onion and parsnips in the olive oil for 3–4 minutes, then add the garlic and dry spices and continue to sauté for another minute. Add the chicken stock and simmer for about 20 minutes or until the parsnip is soft. Blend in a food processor, adding a little more water if the soup is too thick, and reheat. Serve garnished with the chopped coriander.

VARIATION *Prepare with sweet potato, pumpkin or a mixture of root vegetables instead of parsnips.*

DUCK AND EGG NOODLE SOUP
PREPARATION TIME: 10 minutes plus 2 hours marinating and
30 minutes soaking
COOKING TIME: 10–15 minutes

HERBS AND SPICES
4 garlic cloves, crushed
1 green chilli, sliced
Chopped fresh coriander

ALKALINE
4–6 spring onions, sliced
8 dried Chinese or shiitake mushrooms
4 baby bok choy, cut into halves or quarters depending on their
size

NEARLY NEUTRAL
2 tbsp olive oil
1 l chicken stock
2 tsp seasame oil
2 tsp sesame seeds

ACID
2-3 duck breasts, skinned and sliced
2 tbsp light soya sauce
350 g dried egg noodles

Marinate the duck with 1 tablespoon olive oil and the soya
sauce for at least 2 hours. Pour boiling water over the
mushrooms and leave them to soak for 30 minutes. Cook the
noodles in plenty of boiling water according to the
instructions on the packet. Pan-fry the duck in the marinade
until it is thoroughly cooked, reserve and keep warm. While
the duck is cooking, heat the remaining olive oil and sauté the
garlic, spring onions, and chilli for 1 minute. Add the stock
and the mushrooms together with the liquid they have been
soaked in and simmer for about 3-4 minutes. Add the bok
choy and continue to simmer for 2-3 minutes until the bok
choy is just cooked, then add the seasame oil and continue to
simmer for another minute. Divide the noodles among 4
serving bowls, place duck breast slices on the noodles,
sprinkle with the sesame seeds and coriander and ladle over
the soup and vegetables. Serve with additional soya sauce to
taste.

RED PEPPER AND CELERY SOUP
PREPARATION TIME: 10 minutes
COOKING TIME: 20 minutes

HERBS AND SPICES
4-5 cloves garlic, sliced
1 red chilli or to taste
Pepper to taste
Fresh parsley or coriander

ALKALINE
2 medium onions, chopped
3 red peppers, seeded and chopped
3–4 sticks celery, coarsely chopped

NEARLY NEUTRAL
3 tbsp olive oil
1¼ l vegetable stock

Heat the olive oil, add the onion and sauté for 3–4 minutes.
Add the garlic, chilli, red peppers and celery and sauté for
another 2–3 minutes. Add the stock, bring to a slow simmer,
cover and cook gently for about 10–15 minutes until the
vegetables are soft. Purée with a hand blender or using a food
processor and season to taste. Serve garnished with the
coriander or parsley.

VARIATION Use 2 medium zucchini instead of the celery.

SIMPLE MISO SOUP WITH SPINACH AND PRAWNS
PREPARATION TIME: 1 minute
COOKING TIME: 5 minutes

HERBS AND SPICES
Chopped fresh coriander

ALKALINE
60 g baby spinach leaves
4 spring onions, finely sliced

NEARLY NEUTRAL
4 sachets instant miso soup
5 cups boiling water

ACID
16 green prawns
2 tbsp miso paste

Divide the raw spinach leaves and spring onions among 4 serving bowls. Empty the contents of the miso sachets into a saucepan, cover with boiling water and stir to dissolve the soup powder. Add the green prawns and simmer the soup for 2–3 minutes until the prawns have just turned pink. Remove the soup from the heat, put the miso paste in a small sieve and lower into the soup and stir until the miso is dissolved, discarding any left undissolved in the sieve. Divide the prawns between the bowls and pour over the soup. Serve garnished with chopped coriander.

VARIATION Use silken tofu instead of prawns.

VEGETABLE NOODLE SOUP
PREPARATION TIME: 10 minutes
COOKING TIME: 5–6 minutes

HERBS AND SPICES
3–4 cloves garlic, chopped
½ large red chilli, chopped
½ cup chopped fresh coriander leaves

ALKALINE
4 large shiitake mushrooms, cut into pieces
80 g snow peas
80 g bamboo shoots
3–4 spring onions sliced

NEARLY NEUTRAL
1¼ l chicken stock
1 tbsp rice wine or mirin

ACID
125 g rice vermicelli noodles
60 g baby corn
1½ tbsp soya sauce

Pour boiling water over the rice noodles and leave them to stand for 3–5 minutes, then drain and keep warm. Bring the stock to a gentle simmer, add the garlic, chilli, corn and mushrooms and continue to simmer gently for 4–5 minutes. Add the snow peas, bamboo shoots, spring onions, soya sauce and rice wine to the stock and continue to simmer for another minute. Divide the noodles among 4 serving bowls and pour over the soup. Serve garnished with the coriander.

VARIATION
● *Add sliced cooked chicken to the snow peas, bamboo shoots and spring onions.*
● *Add uncooked prawns to the garlic, chilli, corn and mushrooms.*
● *Add cubed bean curd to the snow peas, bamboo shoots and spring onions.*

VICHYSSOISE
PREPARATION TIME: 5 minutes
COOKING TIME: 25 minutes

HERBS AND SPICES
4–5 cloves garlic, chopped
1 sprig fresh thyme
1 bay leaf
2 tbsp chopped fresh chives
Black pepper to taste

ALKALINE
2 leeks, white part only, washed and sliced
1 stick celery
1 small onion
2 large potatoes, peeled and cubed

NEARLY NEUTRAL
2 tbsp olive oil
1 l vegetable stock
2 tbsp soya cream (optional)

Sauté the leeks, celery and onion in the olive oil for 3–4 minutes then add the garlic and continue to sauté for another minute. Add the potatoes and stir to coat with the oil and sauté for another 1–2 minutes. Add the stock, thyme and bay leaf and simmer gently for about 20 minutes or until the potatoes are soft. Remove the herbs, purée the soup (dilute with a little water if too thick), and then chill. Season to taste with freshly ground black pepper and serve garnished with chives and a swirl of soya cream.

NOTE *This soup can be served warm.*

WATERCRESS, SPINACH AND ROCKET SOUP
PREPARATION TIME: 2–3 minutes
COOKING TIME: 10 minutes

HERBS AND SPICES
3–4 cloves garlic, chopped
½–1 large green chilli, chopped
Black pepper to taste

ALKALINE
1 medium brown onion, chopped
100 g mixed watercress, spinach and rocket salad leaves*
180 g baby spinach leaves

NEARLY NEUTRAL
2–3 tbsp olive oil
1 l chicken stock, hot

Heat the oil, add the onion and sauté for 2–3 minutes, then add the garlic and chilli and continue to sauté for another minute. Add the spinach, and mixed spinach, watercress and rocket and stir to coat them with the oil. Add the hot stock and simmer for about 5–6 minutes. Purée using a food processor, and reheat. Season to taste with black pepper.

* *use watercress or rocket alone if a bag of mixed leaves is not available.*

SALADS, SNACKS AND STARTERS

ASIAN NOODLE AND WATERCRESS SALAD

PREPARATION TIME: 5 minutes
COOKING TIME: 3–5 minutes

HERBS AND SPICES
$\frac{1}{2}$ cup fresh coriander, chopped
1 tbsp grated ginger

ALKALINE
150 g mixed watercress and baby spinach leaves
100 g tinned bamboo shoots
5–6 water chestnuts, sliced
4–6 spring onions, sliced
2 tbsp lemon juice

NEARLY NEUTRAL
1 cup bean sprouts
2 tbsp olive oil
2 tbsp sesame oil
2 tbsp mirin

ACID
200 g fresh soba or wonton noodles
2 tbsp light soya sauce
2 tbsp sesame seeds, toasted, or Furikake seasoning*

Cook the noodles in plenty of boiling water following the instructions on the packet. Drain, rinse under cold water, cut into pieces and put in a salad bowl. Add the spinach, watercress, bamboo shoots, water chestnuts, spring onions, bean sprouts and fresh coriander to the noodles. Shake together the ginger, lemon juice, olive oil, sesame oil, mirin and soya sauce, pour over the salad and toss to mix well. Serve sprinkled with the sesame seeds.

* *available from some supermarkets and Asian food shops.*

VARIATION Use fresh egg noodles or spaghetti instead of soba noodles.

AVOCADO AND STRAWBERRY SALAD
PREPARATION TIME: 5 minutes

ALKALINE
2 avocados, stoned and cubed
250 g strawberries, halved
1 tbsp lemon juice
Mixed salad leaves

NEARLY NEUTRAL
2 tbsp olive oil

ACID
1 tbsp balsamic vinegar

Gently mix the avocados and strawberries together. Prepare a dressing by shaking together the olive oil, balsamic vinegar and lemon juice. Pour the dressing over the avocados and strawberries. Serve on a bed of mixed salad leaves.

AVOCADO WITH GINGER PRAWNS
PREPARATION TIME: 5 minutes plus marinating time
COOKING TIME: 3–4 minutes

HERBS AND SPICES
1 tbsp ginger, grated
Chopped fresh coriander

ALKALINE
Mixed salad leaves
2 avocados, peeled, stoned and thickly sliced
1 tbsp lemon juice

NEARLY NEUTRAL
1 tbsp sesame oil

2 tbsp mirin or Chinese rice wine

ACID
2 tbsp light soya sauce
200 g raw large tiger prawns

Mix together the ginger, sesame oil, mirin and soya sauce in a
bowl, add the prawns, stir to coat them in the marinade and set
aside for 1–2 hours. Divide the mixed salad leaves among four
plates. Sprinkle the avocado with a little lemon juice and place
on the lettuce. Heat a small pan or wok, add the prawns with
the marinade and cook for 3–4 minutes until the prawns turn
pink (being careful not to overcook them). Divide the prawns
among the four plates, and pour over the marinade. Serve
garnished with the coriander.

AVOCADO WITH GINGER VINAIGRETTE
PREPARATION TIME: 5–6 minutes

HERBS AND SPICES
2 cloves garlic, crushed
1 tsp fresh ginger, grated
Black pepper

ALKALINE
2 avocados, stoned and halved
2 tbsp lemon juice
Mixed lettuce leaves (optional)

NEARLY NEUTRAL
2 tbsp olive oil

ACID
1 tbsp cider vinegar

Sprinkle the avocados with a little lemon juice to prevent
discolouring. Mix together the olive oil, cider vinegar, garlic,
ginger, remaining lemon juice and black pepper. Place the

avocado on a few mixed lettuce leaves and pour the dressing
into the hole in the avocado.

BEETROOT AND ORANGE SALAD
PREPARATION TIME: 10 minutes
COOKING TIME: 40–50 minutes

HERBS AND SPICES
Black pepper

ALKALINE
4 small beetroot, washed and trimmed
150 g baby spinach leaves
2 small oranges, peeled, segmented and cut in half
1 tbsp lemon juice

NEARLY NEUTRAL
2 tbsp olive oil
12–16 asparagus spears

ACID
2 tbsp walnuts, chopped
1 tbsp walnut oil
2 tbsp red-wine vinegar

Preheat the oven to 180°C. Wrap the beetroot in foil and roast
for 40–50 minutes until cooked, then cool, peel and cut into
slices. Steam or boil the asparagus for 3–4 minutes until just
cooked, then drain and rinse under cold water and cut it into
slices. Mix together the spinach leaves, beetroot, oranges,
asparagus and walnuts in a salad bowl. Shake together the olive
oil, walnut oil, vinegar, lemon juice and black pepper, pour
over the salad and toss to mix well.

VARIATION Use mixed salad leaves instead of baby spinach.

CHICKPEA AND CITRUS CHICKEN SALAD

This recipe was given to us by Chris Williams.
PREPARATION TIME: 5 minutes
COOKING TIME: 30 minutes

HERBS AND SPICES
2 cloves garlic, crushed
1 tbsp Dijon mustard
1 tsp black pepper
4 tbsp chopped fresh mint

ALKALINE
½ cup fresh orange juice
2 tbsp lemon juice
1 cucumber, cut into 1 cm cubes
1 small red Spanish onion, chopped
4 spring onions, sliced
½ green pepper, finely chopped
½ cup raisins or sultanas
100 g mixed salad greens

NEARLY NEUTRAL
2 tbsp soya yoghurt
1 tbsp olive oil

ACID
3 chicken breasts, skinned
1 can chickpeas, drained and rinsed

In a large pan, cover the chicken breasts in cold water and
bring to the boil. Immediately the water boils remove the pan
from the heat, cover and leave to stand for half an hour, then
drain, cool and cut into slices. In a large bowl whisk together
the orange and lemon juices, garlic, yoghurt, mustard and
pepper, then add the olive oil and continue to hand-whisk until
well blended (do not use a food processor). Mix together the
chicken, chickpeas, cucumber, onions, green pepper and
raisins, pour over the dressing and toss to mix well. Divide the

salad greens among the individual plates, add the chicken mixture and sprinkle with mint.

CITRUS SALSA
This recipe was given to us by Chris Williams.
PREPARATION TIME: 15 minutes

HERBS AND SPICES
$\frac{1}{2}$ cup chopped fresh coriander
1 small green chilli, finely sliced (optional)

ALKALINE
1 navel orange, peeled and chopped
1 pink or red grapefruit, peeled, sectioned and chopped
2 slices fresh pineapple, cored and diced
1 medium red onion, chopped
1 red pepper, seeded and chopped
$\frac{1}{2}$ green pepper, seeded and chopped
1 tbsp lemon juice

ACID
1 tbsp balsamic vinegar
2 tbsp olive oil

Mix the fruit, vegetables and herbs together and chill. Just before serving, shake together the lemon juice, vinegar and olive oil, pour over the salsa and stir to mix well. Serve with grilled meat or fish or with a curry.

TIP The easiest way to section a grapefruit is to cut it in half and use a grapefruit knife to cut out the grapefruit segments.

CRAB AND CUCUMBER SALAD
PREPARATION TIME: 15 minutes

HERBS AND SPICES
1 red chilli, chopped (or to taste)
2 tbsp chopped coriander or wide-leaved parsley

2 tsp chopped mint
2 garlic cloves, crushed

ALKALINE
$\frac{1}{2}$ cucumber, finely chopped
1 stalk celery, finely sliced
$\frac{1}{2}$ fennel bulb finely chopped
3–4 water chestnuts, finely chopped (optional)
4–6 spring onions, finely sliced
2 tbsp lemon juice
80–100 g mixed salad leaves

NEARLY NEUTRAL
2–3 tbsp olive oil
1 tsp Thai fish sauce

ACID
2 × 170 cans white crabmeat, rinsed and drained

Place the crabmeat in a bowl and break it up with a fork. Add the cucumber, celery, fennel, water chestnuts, spring onions, chilli, mint and coriander and mix together well. Shake together the olive oil, fish sauce, lemon juice, and garlic and pour over the salad. Serve on a bed of mixed salad leaves.

VARIATION Replace half the crab with chopped cooked prawns.

CRISPY GREEN SALAD
PREPARATION TIME: 10 minutes

HERBS AND SPICES
$\frac{1}{2}$ cup coriander leaves

ALKALINE
100–150 g romaine lettuce, torn into pieces
2 stalks celery, sliced
$\frac{1}{2}$ green pepper, seeded and diced
$\frac{1}{2}$ cucumber, chopped into cubes

4–5 spring onions, sliced
2 green apples, cored and cut into cubes
1 cup green grapes, halved
1 tbsp lemon juice

NEARLY NEUTRAL
2 tbsp olive oil

ACID
1 tbsp cider vinegar
1 tbsp soya sauce

Shake together the olive oil, vinegar, soya sauce and lemon juice. Mix together all the prepared salad vegetables, fruit and coriander, pour over the dressing and toss to mix well.

CURRIED RED LENTIL SALAD
PREPARATION TIME: 5 minutes
COOKING TIME: 20 minutes plus cooling time

HERBS AND SPICES
3–4 cloves garlic, crushed
$\frac{1}{2}$ tsp cumin powder
$\frac{1}{2}$ tsp turmeric
$\frac{1}{2}$ tsp coriander powder
$\frac{1}{4}$ tsp cayenne pepper
$\frac{1}{4}$ tsp ground cloves
$\frac{1}{4}$ tsp cinnamon powder
1 cup wide-leaved fresh parsley or coriander, chopped

ALKALINE
1 small red onion, finely chopped
$\frac{1}{2}$ cup raisins
1 red or green pepper, seeded and finely chopped
1 tbsp lemon juice

NEARLY NEUTRAL
3 tbsp olive oil

1 cup water

ACID
1 cup red lentils
1 tbsp Furikake seasoning (available from some supermarkets)

Heat the olive oil and sauté the garlic for one minute. Add all
the dry spices and continue to sauté for another minute. Add
the lentils and stir to coat them well in the spice mix. Add
the water and simmer the lentils gently, uncovered, for
about 12–15 minutes until they are cooked but still slightly
crunchy (add a little more water if necessary). Remove the
lentils from the heat and when they are cool stir through the
onion, pepper, raisins and parsley or coriander. Gently stir in
the lemon juice, sprinkle with Furikake seasoning and if
necessary stir in a little more olive oil and lemon juice. Keep
at room temperature. Serve with other salads or with a
vegetable curry.

FENNEL, CUCUMBER AND SOYA YOGHURT SALAD
PREPARATION TIME: 5–10 minutes

HERBS AND SPICES
2 garlic cloves, crushed
2–3 tbsp fresh mint, finely chopped

ALKALINE
½ fennel bulb, finely chopped
½ cucumber, seeded and finely chopped
4 spring onions, finely sliced
1 tbsp lemon juice

NEARLY NEUTRAL
1–2 cups soya yoghurt

Mix together all the ingredients, and serve as a dip with
vegetables, with other salads or with a curry dish.

GRAPEFRUIT AND SPINACH SALAD
PREPARATION TIME: 10 minutes

HERBS AND SPICES
2 tbsp chopped fresh coriander leaves
2 tbsp chopped chives

ALKALINE
1 red or pink grapefruit
1 large ripe avocado, peeled, stoned and thinly sliced
100 g baby spinach leaves
½ red pepper, thinly sliced
4–6 spring onions, finely sliced
2 tbsp grapefruit juice

NEARLY NEUTRAL
1 tbsp sesame oil

ACID
1 tbsp light soya sauce
1 tbsp Japanese seasoning (Furikake)*

Peel and segment the grapefruit, reserving any juice (see tip page 197). Toss the avocado slices in the grapefruit juice. Put the spinach in a salad bowl, add the grapefruit segments, avocado with the grapefruit juice in which it has been tossed, red pepper, spring onions, coriander and chopped chives. Shake together the soya sauce and sesame oil and pour over the salad. Add the seasoning and toss to mix all the ingredients. This is delicious served with roasted sweet potatoes (page 261) and chicken teriyaki (page 234).

Furikake seasoning is available from some supermarkets and Asian food shops. It can be replaced with mixed black and white sesame seeds.

VARIATIONS Use watercress or rocket instead of spinach or a mixture of all three.

MIXED WATERCRESS, ROCKET, SPINACH AND ZUCCHINI SALAD
PREPARATION TIME: 10 minutes

HERBS AND SPICES
2 tbsp chopped fresh coriander leaves
2 tbsp chopped fresh chives
1 tsp chilli sambal (optional)

ALKALINE
150 g mixed baby spinach, watercress and rocket leaves
2 small zucchini, scrubbed and thinly sliced
4–6 spring onions, finely sliced
1 tbsp lime or lemon juice

NEARLY NEUTRAL
2 tbsp olive oil
1 tsp sesame oil
2 tbsp mirin
1 tbsp sesame seeds

ACID
2 tbsp light soya sauce

Put the spinach, watercress and rocket into a salad bowl, add the zucchini, spring onions, coriander and chives. Shake together the olive oil, sesame oil, mirin, soya sauce, chilli sambal and lime juice and pour over the salad. Toss to mix all the ingredients together and serve sprinkled with the sesame seeds.

VARIATION *This could be made with just watercress, rocket or spinach.*

POTATO SALAD WITH SERGIO'S HOME-MADE MAYONNAISE
PREPARATION TIME: 5 minutes
COOKING TIME: 25 minutes

HERBS AND SPICES
3–4 tbsp chopped chives
5–6 cloves garlic, crushed

ALKALINE
500 g baby salad potatoes
3–4 spring onions, finely sliced
1 tbsp lemon juice

NEARLY NEUTRAL
1 cup olive oil
$^1/_2$ cup sunflower oil

ACID
2 eggs

Boil or steam the potatoes until cooked, cut into large cubes and toss with the spring onions and chives. Lightly beat the eggs and add the garlic. Using a blender, continuously beat the eggs while very slowly adding the olive oil in a steady stream followed by the sunflower oil to form a thick mayonnaise and then add the lemon juice. Add the mayonnaise to the potatoes and mix well

SALMON AND CUCUMBER OPEN SANDWICHES

Salmon bones are an excellent source of calcium, but if you eat the salmon with mayonnaise and 2 slices of bread, the meal may be too acid. We suggest that instead you make an open sandwich using one slice of bread and pile on the cucumber, tomato and herbs.
PREPARATION TIME: 5 minutes

HERBS AND SPICES
$^1/_4$ cup chopped dill
Black pepper

ALKALINE
$^1/_2$–1 cucumber, washed and thinly sliced
2–3 tomatoes, sliced

ACID
350 kg can salmon with bones
4 slices of bread

Drain the salmon, remove the skin and mash the fish and
bones together, and spread on the bread. Top with the sliced
cucumber and tomato, season with ground black pepper and
sprinkle with dill.

SPICY AUBERGINE PURÉE
PREPARATION TIME: 5 minutes
COOKING TIME: 35 minutes

HERBS AND SPICES
3–4 cloves garlic, crushed
1 tbsp ginger, grated
1 tsp cumin powder
$1/2$ tsp cayenne pepper
Fresh coriander and/or mint, chopped

ALKALINE
1 large aubergine
1 tbsp lemon juice
1 small onion, chopped
4 spring onions, finely sliced

NEARLY NEUTRAL
3 tbsp olive oil

Preheat the oven to 220°C. Roast the aubergine for about 30
minutes or until soft. Cool, peel and purée with the lemon
juice in a food processor. Heat the olive oil and fry the onion
for 3–4 minutes, then add the garlic, ginger, cumin and
cayenne pepper and continue to sauté for another minute. Add
the puréed aubergine and sauté for a further two minutes. Stir
through the spring onions and season to taste. Serve garnished
with the coriander and/or mint.

THAI-STYLE CHICKEN NOODLE SALAD
PREPARATION TIME: 5 minutes
COOKING TIME: 5 minutes

HERBS AND SPICES
½ cup mixed coriander and mint, finely chopped
2 lime leaves, sliced very finely
1 small red chilli or 1 tsp chilli sambal

ALKALINE
4 spring onions, finely sliced
12–16 snow peas, sliced
Juice of 2 limes or 1 lemon

NEARLY NEUTRAL
2 tbsp olive oil
1 cup bean sprouts
1 tbsp sesame oil
2 tsp fish sauce

ACID
2 chicken breasts, skinned and sliced
100 g rice vermicelli noodles

Heat the olive oil and stir-fry the chicken until it is thoroughly cooked (about 3–4 minutes). Soak the noodles in boiling water for 2–3 minutes until they are soft, then rinse under cold water and drain. Mix together the chicken, mint and coriander, lime leaves, spring onions, bean sprouts, snow peas and noodles. Shake together the sesame oil, fish sauce, chilli and lime juice. Pour the dressing over the salad, toss and serve immediately.

THAI-STYLE CHICKEN WITH CARROT AND CABBAGE SALAD
PREPARATION TIME: 10 minutes plus 30 minutes to set aside ·
  the dressing
COOKING TIME: 10 minutes

HERBS AND SPICES
3–4 cloves garlic, crushed
1 tbsp chilli sambal
½ cup fresh mint, chopped
½ cup fresh coriander, chopped

ALKALINE
1 cup green cabbage, grated or finely shredded
1 cup red cabbage, grated or finely shredded
1 cup carrot, grated
½ fennel, grated or finely shredded
1 medium red onion, finely sliced
4–6 spring onions, sliced
3 tbsp fresh lime or lemon juice

NEARLY NEUTRAL
1 cup bean sprouts
2 tbsp olive oil
2 tbsp sesame oil
2 tsp fish sauce

ACID
2 chicken breasts
1 tbsp rice vinegar

Shake together the garlic, lime juice, vinegar, fish sauce, oils and chilli and leave for at least half an hour. Poach the chicken (as described on page 216) or use left-over chicken cut into slices. Mix together all the salad ingredients and the mint and coriander, add the chicken, pour over the dressing and toss to mix well.

WILD RICE SALAD
PREPARATION TIME: 15 minutes
COOKING TIME: 30–40 minutes

HERBS AND SPICES
2 cloves garlic, crushed
2 tbsp fresh parsley

Black pepper

ALKALINE
1 red onion, chopped
½ fennel bulb, thinly sliced
1 Granny Smith apple, finely sliced
½ cucumber, chopped
1 stick celery, finely sliced
1 tbsp lemon juice
½ cup raisins

NEARLY NEUTRAL
2 tbsp sunflower oil
3 cups water
3 tbsp olive oil

ACID
1 cup wild rice
½ cup pine nuts
1 tbsp white wine vinegar

Heat the sunflower oil and sauté the onion for 2–3 minutes,
add the garlic and rice and continue to sauté for another
minute. Add the water, season to taste, cover and simmer
gently for about 30–40 minutes until the rice is cooked. Drain
the rice and rinse under cold water. Add the fennel, apple,
cucumber, celery, pine nuts, raisins and parsley to the rice and
mix together. Shake together the olive oil, white wine vinegar
and lemon juice, pour over the salad and toss.

VARIATION *Use half wild rice and half basmati rice.*

Salad suggestions
Grated carrot, zucchini and celery salad
Avocado and apple salad
Mushroom, zucchini and snow pea salad

GREAT GRAINS AND MEAN BEANS

All grains and legumes, including beans, contain protein and are therefore acid forming to some degree. They should be balanced with vegetables, and ideally eaten separately from other acid-forming foods such as meat.

TIP PERFECT RICE With basmati or long-grain rice add 2 cups of water to the first cup of rice and one cup of water for each additional cup of rice. For Japanese-style, short grained rice, allow 1½ cups of water for the first cup of rice and one cup of water for each additional cup. Rinse the rice, and add to a saucepan of cold water. Bring to the boil, reduce to a gentle simmer, cover and leave to cook gently until all the water is absorbed (about 15 minutes). The rice can be fried in a little olive oil for a few minutes before adding the water, which gives it more flavour.

BEAN CURD ROLLS

We have recently found fresh bean curd sheets in our local Chinese supermarket. They make a delicious alternative to spring rolls.

PREPARATION TIME: 20 minutes
COOKING TIME: 10 minutes
HERBS AND SPICES
2 red chillies, sliced lengthways
Fresh chives, chopped
Fresh coriander, chopped sprigs

ALKALINE
100 g canned bamboo shoots, rinsed and drained
1 carrot
2 spring onions
8 snow peas
½ red or green pepper

NEARLY NEUTRAL
3 tbsp peanut oil

100 g bean sprouts
1 tsp sesame oil

ACID
1 tbsp light soya sauce or Thai chilli dipping sauce
1 packet bean curd sheets

Cut the bamboo shoots, carrot, snow peas, red pepper and spring onions into thin strips of about the same length as the bean sprouts. Heat the peanut oil and stir-fry the vegetables and chilli for 2 minutes. Add the chives, fresh coriander, sesame oil and soya sauce, stir well, continuing to stir-fry for another minute, then remove from the heat, drain any excess liquid and leave to cool. Cut the bean curd sheet into squares, place about 2 tbsp of the vegetable mix on each square, add some chives and fresh coriander, and roll to make a neat parcel. Seal the edges with a little thick paste made from flour and water. Fry the bean curd rolls in hot oil for about 3–4 minutes. Serve with soya sauce or Thai chilli dipping sauce.

VARIATION Use rice paper wrappers.

BEAN CURD WITH OYSTER SAUCE
PREPARATION TIME: 5 minutes
COOKING TIME: 10 minutes

HERBS AND SPICES
3–4 cloves garlic, crushed
1 tbsp ginger, grated
1 red chilli, sliced
$\frac{1}{2}$ cup fresh coriander, chopped

ALKALINE
3 sticks of celery sliced
6 spring onions, sliced
1 red pepper, diced
125 g fresh shiitake, oyster or baby mushrooms, sliced

NEARLY NEUTRAL
2 tbsp olive oil
$\frac{1}{2}$ cup water
2 tbsp oyster sauce
1 tbsp mirin or Chinese cooking wine

ACID
250 g bean curd or tofu cut into cubes
1 tbsp soya sauce

Heat the olive oil and fry the bean curd for about 3–4 minutes
or until it has turned a light brown colour, tossing occasionally,
then remove from the pan and keep warm. Add the garlic,
ginger and chilli to the pan and stir-fry for one minute then
add the celery, pepper, spring onions and mushrooms, stir to
coat in the oil and continue to stir-fry for 1–2 minutes. Add the
water, oyster sauce, mirin and soya sauce, bring to a gentle
simmer, cover and stir-fry for 1–2 minutes until the vegetables
are just tender. Add the bean curd to the vegetables, toss gently
and heat through. Serve garnished with coriander.

CHICKPEAS WITH MOROCCAN AUBERGINE
PREPARATION TIME: 10 minutes
COOKING TIME: 15 minutes

HERBS AND SPICES
4–6 cloves garlic, crushed
1 red chilli, chopped or 1 tsp cayenne pepper
2 tsp ground coriander
2 tsp ground cumin
1 tsp paprika
$\frac{1}{2}$ cup fresh coriander, chopped
2 tbsp fresh mint, chopped

ALKALINE
1 red onion, chopped
1 medium aubergine, cut into 1 cm cubes
4–5 medium vine-ripened tomatoes, chopped

4 tbsp lemon juice

NEARLY NEUTRAL
3 tbsp olive oil
Soya yoghurt

ACID
1 can chickpeas, rinsed and drained
Pitta bread

Heat the oil and sauté the onion for 2–3 minutes then add the garlic, chilli and dry spices and continue to sauté for another minute. Add the aubergine, tomatoes and lemon juice and simmer gently for 5–10 minutes. Add the chickpeas and simmer for another 5 minutes. Stir in the coriander and mint, pour into a serving dish and leave to cool to room temperature. Serve with some soya yoghurt and pitta bread.

COUSCOUS WITH ASPARAGUS AND PEAS
PREPARATION TIME: 5 minutes
COOKING TIME: 6 minutes

HERBS AND SPICES
3–4 garlic cloves, crushed
Black pepper
Torn fresh basil leaves

ALKALINE
16 snow peas, halved
4 spring onions, sliced

NEARLY NEUTRAL
2 tbsp olive oil
8 stalks asparagus, cut into 4 pieces
2½ cups vegetable or chicken stock
1 tbsp sesame seeds

ACID
2 cups couscous
1 cup frozen peas

Heat the stock, pour it over the couscous and leave to stand for
about 5–6 minutes or according to the instructions on the
packet. Heat the olive oil and sauté the garlic and asparagus for
about 1 minute, add a little water, cover and sauté for another 3
minutes. Add the snow peas, spring onions, and peas and
continue to cook for another 1–2 minutes until the peas are
warmed through (if using fresh peas, add to the olive oil about
five minutes before the asparagus). Stir the vegetables through
the couscous. Season with pepper and serve sprinkled with
sesame seeds and basil.

COUSCOUS WITH SALMON AND CUCUMBER
PREPARATION TIME: 5 minutes
COOKING TIME: 5 minutes

HERBS AND SPICES
1 cup fresh parsley or coriander, chopped
Black pepper

ALKALINE
1 cucumber, finely chopped
2 tomatoes, finely chopped
1 small red onion, finely chopped
2 tbsp lemon juice
Mixed salad leaves

NEARLY NEUTRAL
2½ cups vegetable or chicken stock or hot water
3 tbsp olive oil

ACID
2 cups couscous
400 g canned red salmon with bones, drained

Pour the hot stock over the couscous, season to taste, cover and leave to stand for 5–6 minutes. Break up the salmon and the bones with a fork, removing any large bits of skin. Add the salmon, cucumber, tomato, onion and parsley or coriander to the couscous and mix well with a fork and season to taste. Mix together the oil and lemon juice and pour over the couscous. Serve on a bed of mixed salad leaves.

FRIED TOFU WITH SESAME SEEDS
PREPARATION TIME: 5 minutes
COOKING TIME: 10–20 minutes

NEARLY NEUTRAL
¼ cup groundnut or sunflower oil for frying

ACID
250 g firm tofu
¼ cup plain flour
1 egg, lightly beaten
2 tbsp Furikake Japanese seasoning

Press the tofu between two boards to remove any excess moisture. Cut the tofu into cubes, toss them in flour, dip them into the egg and then coat them with Furikake seasoning. Heat the oil in a wok and cook the tofu in batches until lightly browned all over.

HUMMUS
Hummus is a great staple and although acid generating, if served with a baked potato gives a well-balanced snack or meal.
PREPARATION TIME: 2 minutes
(and overnight if using dried chickpeas)
COOKING TIME: 1–2 hours if using dried chickpeas

HERBS AND SPICES
4 cloves garlic
1 tsp paprika

ALKALINE
3 tbsp lemon juice

NEARLY NEUTRAL
1 tbsp olive oil
⅓ cup tahini
¼–½ cup of water

ACID
1 can chickpeas or 175 g dried chickpeas soaked overnight and
  boiled in fresh water for 1–2 hours

Add the chickpeas, garlic, tahini and lemon juice to a food
processor or blender and gradually add the water until the
hummus reaches a smooth creamy consistency. Season to taste.
Put in a bowl, pour over a little olive oil on the surface and
sprinkle with paprika.

LEEK, PEA AND ASPARAGUS RISOTTO
PREPARATION TIME: 5 minutes
COOKING TIME: 30 minutes

HERBS AND SPICES
4 cloves garlic, crushed
½ tsp turmeric or saffron
Black pepper
½ cup fresh basil leaves

ALKALINE
½ onion, sliced
2 leeks, washed and finely sliced
1 tbsp lemon juice

NEARLY NEUTRAL
2 tbsp olive oil
8 asparagus stalks, sliced into 1 cm lengths
500 ml chicken stock

ACID
1 cup fresh or frozen peas
1 cup risotto rice

Heat the stock to a gentle simmer. In a separate pan, sauté the
onion and leek in the olive oil for 3–4 minutes until they are
transparent, then add the garlic and continue to stauté for
another minute. Add the rice, peas, asparagus and turmeric,
stirring until the rice is well coated with the oil and turmeric.
Slowly add the chicken stock, a cup at a time, stirring
continuously until the rice is cooked. You may need to slightly
adjust the quantity of stock to ensure the rice is cooked
through but not too moist. Season with black pepper to taste,
stir through the lemon juice and torn basil leaves and serve
immediately.

PASTA AND CHICKEN SALAD
PREPARATION TIME: 10 minutes
COOKING TIME: 10 minutes

HERBS AND SPICES
½ cup fresh coriander, coarsely chopped
½ cup fresh mint, coarsely chopped
1 tsp chilli sambal or 1 red chilli, chopped

ALKALINE
8 cherry tomatoes, cut into quarters
¾ cucumber, chopped
½ red or green pepper, seeded and cut into cubes
12 snow peas, halved
4–6 spring onions, sliced
2 tbsp lemon juice

NEARLY NEUTRAL
1 cup bean sprouts
1 tbsp sesame oil
2 tsp fish sauce
1 tbsp mirin

ACID
200 g dry pasta such as spiralli
2 chicken breasts, skinned
1 tbsp soya sauce

Cook the pasta in plenty of boiling water following the instructions on the packet, drain and rinse with cold water. If using long noodles, chop them coarsely. Poach the chicken breasts for about 10 minutes or until they are just cooked through, then drain and cut them into thin slices. Mix together all the salad ingredients, mint, coriander and chicken. Shake together the chilli sambal, sesame oil, soya sauce, fish sauce, mirin and lemon juice, pour over the salad and toss gently to mix well.

PASTA WITH PRAWNS AND PEAS

This dish is acid-generating, so serve it with green salad or after a vegetable soup.
PREPARATION TIME: 5 minutes
COOKING TIME: 10 minutes

HERBS AND SPICES
3–4 cloves garlic, crushed
1 green chilli, chopped
$\frac{1}{2}$ cup fresh coriander or Italian parsley, coarsely chopped
Black pepper

ALKALINE
100 g snow peas
4–5 spring onions, sliced
1 tbsp lemon juice

NEARLY NEUTRAL
3 tbsp olive oil
$\frac{1}{2}$ cup dry white wine or vegetable stock

ACID
200 g penne

250 g prawns, peeled
1 cup frozen peas

Cook the pasta in plenty of boiling water following the instructions on the packet and drain. While the pasta is cooking, heat the olive oil in a wok or sauté pan and stir-fry the garlic and chilli for about 10 seconds. Add the wine or stock and simmer for 5 minutes. Add the prawns and continue to simmer until they turn pink. Add the peas, snow peas and spring onions and cook for a further 1–2 minutes. Stir through the lemon juice, coriander or parsley and season to taste with black pepper and sauté for another minute. Divide the pasta among 4 serving plates and top with the prawn mixture. Serve immediately.

PIZZA WITH OLIVE PASTE AND SAUTÉED PEPPERS

A pizza bought from a takeaway is almost always acid-generating, especially if it contains cheese. This is a simple, delicious and well-balanced alternative.
PREPARATION TIME: 10 minutes
COOKING TIME: 30 minutes

HERBS AND SPICES
6 garlic cloves, chopped
2 long red chillies, chopped
½ cup torn fresh basil leaves
Pepper to taste

ALKALINE
1 red onion, sliced
4 mixed peppers, seeded and thinly sliced
16 vine-ripened cherry tomatoes, halved
1 cup olive paste (page 172)

NEARLY NEUTRAL
3–4 tbsp olive oil

ACID
1 pizza base
2 tbsp balsamic vinegar

Heat the olive oil, add the onion and peppers and fry for about 10 minutes. Add the garlic, tomatoes, balsamic vinegar and chilli and sauté for a further 15 minutes. Spread the pizza base with olive paste, top with the vegetables and sprinkle with basil. Cook the pizza in a preheated 220°C oven for about 15 minutes or until pizza base is golden brown on the edges.

RICE NOODLES WITH CHILLI PRAWNS AND SNOW PEAS
PREPARATION TIME: 5 minutes
COOKING TIME: 5 minutes

HERBS AND SPICES
2–3 cloves garlic, sliced
2 tsp chilli sambal
$\frac{1}{2}$ cup fresh mint, chopped
$\frac{1}{2}$ cup fresh coriander, chopped

ALKALINE
400 g snow peas, sliced
3–4 spring onions, sliced
2 tbsp lemon juice

NEARLY NEUTRAL
2 tbsp olive oil
1 tbsp fish sauce

ACID
125 g rice vermicelli noodles
250 g peeled green prawns

Put the noodles in a bowl, cover with boiling water and leave to stand for 5–6 minutes or cook according to the instructions on the packet. Heat the olive oil and sauté the garlic and chilli sambal for one minute. Add the prawns and stir-fry for 3–4 minutes until they become pink. Add the snow peas, spring onions, fish sauce and lemon juice and continue to stir-fry for another 1–2 minutes, then stir through the mint and coriander. Divide the noodles among the plates and top with the chilli prawns and snow peas.

SESAME BEAN CURD WITH SNOW PEAS AND ALMONDS

This recipe was given to us by Diana Lampe.
PREPARATION TIME: 10 minutes plus 1 hour marinating
COOKING TIME: 10 minutes

HERBS AND SPICES
2 cloves garlic, crushed
2 tsp grated fresh ginger
1 red chilli, finely chopped
1 cup fresh coriander leaves

ALKALINE
2 cups fresh baby spinach leaves
2 cups snow peas, sliced
6 spring onions, sliced diagonally

NEARLY NEUTRAL
2 tbsp sesame oil
$\frac{1}{2}$ tbsp groundnut oil
1 tbsp sesame seeds

ACID
1 block firm bean curd
2 tbsp light soya sauce
2 tbsp rice vinegar
$\frac{1}{3}$ cup almonds, toasted

Cut the bean curd into 1 cm cubes. Shake together 1 tbsp sesame oil, the soya sauce and crushed garlic, pour over the bean curd and leave to marinate for at least an hour. Fry the bean curd in the marinade for about 8–10 minutes, tossing to ensure it is cooked on all sides. Mix together the spinach, snow peas, spring onions, sesame seeds, almonds, coriander and bean curd. Prepare a dressing with the groundnut oil, remaining sesame oil, rice vinegar, ginger and chilli. Pour over the salad and toss gently.

SPAGHETTI WITH FRESH WILD SALMON AND TOMATOES

Wild salmon is delicious and an excellent source of natural omega 3 oil.
PREPARATION TIME: 10 minutes
COOKING TIME: 10 minutes

HERBS AND SPICES
4–5 cloves garlic, chopped
1 large red chilli, chopped
1 cup fresh wide-leaved parsley, chopped
Black pepper

ALKALINE
1 onion, chopped
3 tbsp small capers, drained
6 medium vine-ripened tomatoes, chopped

NEARLY NEUTRAL
3 tbsp olive oil
½ cup red wine or water

ACID
500 g fresh spaghetti
150 g wild salmon, skinned and cut into cubes

Cook the pasta in plenty of boiling water according to the instructions on the packet and drain. Meanwhile heat the olive oil and sauté the onion for 3–4 minutes, then add the garlic and chilli and continue to sauté for another minute. Add the capers, tomatoes and wine and simmer for 3–4 minutes. Add the salmon and continue to cook for another 3–4 minutes until the salmon is just cooked. Stir through the parsley and season with black pepper. Divide the spaghetti among the plates, top with the salmon and tomato sauce, and serve immediately.

SPAGHETTI WITH ZUCCHINI AND PEAS
PREPARATION TIME: 5 minutes
COOKING TIME: 10 minutes

HERBS AND SPICES
4 cloves garlic, crushed
1 green chilli, chopped (optional)
$\frac{1}{2}$ cup basil leaves
Pepper to taste

ALKALINE
4 medium zucchini, scrubbed and thinly sliced
4–5 spring onions, sliced
2 tbsp lemon juice

NEARLY NEUTRAL
3 tbsp olive oil
$\frac{1}{2}$ cup white wine or chicken stock

ACID
250 g spaghetti or linguine
2 cups frozen or fresh peas

Cook the spaghetti in plenty of boiling water following the instructions on the packet and drain. Heat the olive oil and sauté the garlic and chilli for about 10 seconds. Add the zucchini and peas and continue to sauté for 1–2 minutes. Add the wine or stock and simmer for about 5 minutes until the zucchini is soft. Add the spring onions and basil, stir and simmer for one minute. Add the sautéed vegetables to the pasta, toss to mix well and season with black pepper (a little extra olive oil can be added if there is insufficient liquid to coat the pasta).

SENSUOUS SEAFOOD

All fish and seafood is acid forming, so serve them with plenty of additional vegetables.

BAKED COD WITH LENTILS, TOMATO AND FENNEL

PREPARATION TIME: 5 minutes
COOKING TIME: 40 minutes

HERBS AND SPICES
3–4 garlic cloves, crushed
1 cup fresh coriander or parsley, chopped

ALKALINE
180 g baby spinach leaves
100 g fennel finely chopped
200 g vine-ripened tomatoes, finely chopped

NEARLY NEUTRAL
4 tbsp olive oil
2 cups water

ACID
200 g Puy lentils
500 g cod, skinned, boned and cut into 4 pieces

Preheat the oven to 180°C. Add the lentils to a pan, cover with the water, bring to a boil and then simmer for about 35–40 minutes until the water is absorbed and the lentils are soft. If the lentils dry out before they are cooked just add more water. Put the cod in a baking tray and pour over a little olive oil and bake for 15 minutes. Add 2 tablespoons of the olive oil to a frying pan and gently sauté the fennel for 3–4 minutes until it is soft. Add the garlic and continue to sauté for another minute then add the spinach and tomatoes and sauté until the spinach is just wilted. Mix the vegetables and coriander or parsley through the lentils. Serve the lentils on to plates and top with the baked cod.

VARIATION Poach the cod gently on top of the stove.

BAKED SEA BASS WITH STIR FRIED SPINACH AND FENNEL
PREPARATION TIME: 5 minutes
COOKING TIME: 15–20 minutes

HERBS AND SPICES
4 garlic cloves crushed
1 tsp fresh ginger, grated
2–3 tbsp fresh basil chopped

ALKALINE
2 tbsp lemon juice
1 fennel bulb, finely sliced
4–8 field mushrooms, sliced
200 g baby spinach leaves

NEARLY NEUTRAL
4 tbsp olive oil

ACID
2–4 small to medium sea bass

Preheat the oven to 180°C. Put the sea bass in a baking dish and
drizzle over 2 tablespoons of the olive oil and the lemon juice
and bake for 15–20 minutes or until just cooked. Meanwhile, heat
the remaining olive oil in a sauté pan or wok and stir-fry the
garlic, ginger and fennel for 2–3 minutes, then add the
mushrooms and continue to stir-fry for another 2 minutes. Add
the spinach and stir to coat it well with the oil, cover and
continue to cook until the spinach is just wilted (about 1 minute).
Fillet the sea bass if using less than 4 fish. Divide the vegetables
between four plates, top with the sea bass and sprinkle with basil.

CHILLI PRAWNS
PREPARATION TIME: 5 minutes
COOKING TIME: 6–7 minutes

HERBS AND SPICES
3–4 cloves garlic, crushed
1–2 long red chillies, sliced
1 tbsp ginger, grated
1 tbsp Thai sweet chilli dipping sauce or chilli sauce
3 tbsp coriander, chopped

ALKALINE
1 small onion, chopped
4 spring onions, sliced

NEARLY NEUTRAL
2 tbsp olive oil
$\frac{1}{4}$ cup tomato sauce
2 tbsp mirin or Chinese cooking wine

ACID
500 g green prawns
1 tbsp light soya sauce

Heat the olive oil in a wok and stir-fry the onion for 2–3
minutes, then add the garlic, ginger and chilli and continue to
stir-fry for another minute. Add the tomato, chilli, and soya
sauces and mirin and continue to stir-fry for another minute. If
the sauce is too thick add a little water. Add the prawns, stir to
ensure they are well coated in the sauce, cover the pan, and
continue to stir-fry until the prawns turn pink. Stir through the
coriander and spring onions. Serve with steamed rice and
steamed Chinese vegetables.

VARIATION *Use fresh crab or frozen crab claws (from your Asian
supermarket). Clean the crab and cut it into pieces. Fry the crab
separately and stir it into the chilli sauce.*

FRESH TUNA WITH NORI

PREPARATION TIME: 6–7 minutes
COOKING TIME: 4–5 minutes

HERBS AND SPICES
½ tsp wasabi paste

ALKALINE
2–3 sheets of nori seaweed

ACID
4 tuna steaks (about 400 g)
Tamari or light soya sauce for dipping

Spread a very thin layer of the wasabi paste on one side of the tuna. Wrap the tuna steaks tightly in a single sheet of nori, trimming off any excess. Cook the tuna on a high heat in a griddle pan for 1–2 minutes each side (tuna becomes very tough if it is overcooked and it is best just lightly seared) or until cooked through to your liking. Slice the tuna into thin strips and serve with steamed rice and beans with ginger (page 257) or with a salad and tamari or light soya sauce for dipping.

GRILLED FISH WITH SOYA SAUCE
PREPARATION TIME: 2–3 minutes plus marinating time
COOKING TIME: 5–6 minutes

HERBS AND SPICES
4 cloves garlic, crushed
1 small red chilli, chopped
½ cup fresh coriander, chopped

ALKALINE
2 tsp fresh lime juice

NEARLY NEUTRAL
2 tbsp mirin or Chinese cooking wine

ACID
3 tbsp light soya sauce
4 fillets cod or other firm-fleshed white fish

Blend together the lime juice, garlic, chilli, mirin and soya
sauce in a food processor and pour over the fish fillets and
leave to marinate for about 15 minutes. Bake or pan-fry the
fish with the marinade for about 5–6 minutes until the fish is
just cooked. Serve garnished with coriander. Accompany with
steamed bok choy or any other vegetable dish and baked
sweet potato.

MIXED SEAFOOD STEW

PREPARATION TIME: 5–10 minutes
COOKING TIME: 25–30 minutes

HERBS AND SPICES
4–5 garlic cloves finely chopped
1 red chilli (or to taste)
Chopped coriander or parsley

ALKALINE
1 small red onion, chopped
2 stalks celery, finely chopped
12 cherry tomatoes, chopped
8–10 small mushrooms, halved
12–16 snow peas, halved
2 tbsp lemon juice

NEARLY NEUTRAL
2–3 tbsp olive oil

ACID
500 g fresh mussels in their shells
150 g scallops
150 g green tiger prawns (without shells)
2–3 squid, sliced into rings
4 very large tiger prawns with shells on (optional)

Clean the mussels and rinse all the other seafood in cold
water. Heat the oil and sauté the onion for 2–3 minutes, then
add the garlic and chilli and continue to sauté for another

minute. Add the celery and cook for another 2–3 minutes.
Add the tomatoes, cover and simmer for a further 10 minutes.
Add the mushrooms and the large tiger prawns and simmer
for about 2–3 minutes until the prawns are just pink. Add the
other prawns, mussels and snow peas and cook for another 2
minutes. Add the scallops, squid and lemon juice and
continue to cook for 1–2 minutes (if the squid and scallops
are added too early they will be tough). Serve in bowls and
garnish with coriander or parsley.

SALMON AND SWEET POTATO CAKES

PREPARATION TIME: 15 minutes
COOKING TIME: 20 minutes

HERBS AND SPICES
¼ tsp turmeric
1 red chilli, finely sliced
2 tbsp Italian parsley, finely chopped
2–3 tbsp chives, finely chopped

ALKALINE
1–2 cups coconut milk
250 g sweet potato, peeled and grated

NEARLY NEUTRAL
Sunflower or groundnut oil for frying

ACID
200 g canned red salmon with bones
½ cup self-raising flour
½ cup rice flour

Drain the salmon, remove any large pieces of skin and mash.
Mix together the self-raising and rice flours and turmeric and
gradually add the coconut milk to make a thick batter. Stir in
the sweet potato, salmon, chives, chilli and parsley and mix
well (add more coconut milk if necessary, but be careful not to
make the batter too thin). Heat the oil in a wok and fry

spoonfuls of the salmon and potato mix for 3–4 minutes each side until they are well browned on the outside and cooked through but soft inside. Drain on kitchen paper and serve with Thai chilli dipping sauce.

VARIATION *Use any fish or chopped prawns; replace parsley with coriander or dill.*

SEAFOOD PAELLA
PREPARATION TIME: 10 minutes
COOKING TIME: 30 minutes

HERBS AND SPICES
4–5 cloves garlic, minced
1 red chilli, chopped or to taste
Black pepper
Chopped parsley or coriander

ALKALINE
1 medium onion, sliced
16 snap peas
1 red pepper, seeded and sliced
16 snow peas
12 cherry tomatoes, halved
2 large handfuls (90 g) baby spinach leaves

NEARLY NEUTRAL
2–3 tbsp olive oil
2 cups heated chicken or vegetable stock

ACID
1 cup paella rice, washed and drained
500 g fresh mussels
4 large green prawns (unshelled)
6 small squid, cut into rings
100 g shelled green prawns
100 g small scallops

Heat the olive oil and sauté the onion for 2–3 minutes, add the garlic and chilli and sauté for another minute. Add the rice, stir to coat with the oil and continue to sauté for another minute. Add the stock, cover and simmer gently for about 15 minutes. Then add the snap peas, red pepper, tomatoes and large prawns, cover and simmer for another five minutes. Add the mussels and continue to simmer for another 2–3 minutes, then add the scallops, prawns, squid, snow peas, and spinach, stir to mix well and sauté for another 2–3 minutes until all the seafood is just cooked through and the spinach has wilted. Season with black pepper and serve garnished with chopped parsley or coriander.

SQUID IN SOYA SAUCE
PREPARATION TIME: 5 minutes
COOKING TIME: 5 minutes

HERBS AND SPICES
3–4 cloves garlic, crushed
1 tbsp fresh ginger, grated
½ long red chilli or to taste

NEARLY NEUTRAL
2 tbsp olive oil

ACID
500 g baby squid, washed and cut into rings
1 tbsp light soya sauce

Heat the olive oil and stir-fry the garlic, ginger and chilli for 1 minute. Add the squid and continue to stir-fry for 2–3 minutes. Add the soya sauce and continue to cook for another minute (do not overcook or the squid will be tough).

STIR-FRIED PRAWNS WITH BROCCOLI AND SNOW PEAS
PREPARATION TIME: 5 minutes
COOKING TIME: 12–15 minutes

HERBS AND SPICES
3–4 cloves garlic, crushed
1 tbsp fresh ginger, grated
1 long green chilli, chopped
Fresh coriander

ALKALINE
200 g broccoli, cut into small florets
220 g tinned bamboo shoots or water chestnuts
16 baby mushrooms
60 g snow peas

NEARLY NEUTRAL
2 tbsp olive oil
½ cup chicken stock
1 tbsp oyster sauce

ACID
250 g egg noodles
300 g green prawns

Cook the noodles in plenty of boiling water according to the instructions on the packet. Drain and keep warm. Heat the olive oil and stir-fry the garlic, ginger and chilli for 1 minute. Add the broccoli, stir to ensure it is coated in the oil, then add the chicken stock, cover and simmer for about 3 to 4 minutes. Add the prawns and mushrooms and continue to cook for a further 3–4 minutes until all the prawns are pink. Add the bamboo shoots, snow peas and oyster sauce and cook for another 2 minutes. Divide the noodles between four dishes, top with the prawns and garnish with coriander.

VARIATION *Use scallops or mixed seafood instead of the prawns.*

STIR-FRIED SCALLOPS WITH BOK CHOY AND SNOW PEAS
PREPARATION TIME: 5 minutes plus 20 minutes marinating time

COOKING TIME: 5 minutes

HERBS AND SPICES
1 tbsp fresh ginger, grated
2–3 garlic cloves, crushed

ALKALINE
200 g bok choy
4–6 spring onions, sliced
60 g snow peas

NEARLY NEUTRAL
2 tbsp rice wine
1 tbsp sesame oil
1 tbsp olive oil
⅓ cup chicken stock

ACID
350 g scallops

Mix together the rice wine, ginger and sesame oil, pour over the scallops and marinate for at least 20 minutes. Heat the olive oil and stir-fry the garlic, bok choy and spring onions for 2–3 minutes. Add the scallops, with the marinade, chicken stock and snow peas, cover and cook for 1–2 minutes until the scallops are just cooked.

VARIATION *Use prawns instead of the scallops.*

THAI-STYLE CURRIED COD WITH YELLOW PEPPERS
PREPARATION TIME: 15 minutes
COOKING TIME: 15 minutes

HERBS AND SPICES
7–8 garlic cloves
2.5 cm ginger
2–3 red chillies

4 stalks lemon grass, cut into 5 cm pieces and slightly crushed
6 lime leaves
2 tbsp turmeric
$\frac{1}{2}$ cup fresh coriander, chopped

ALKALINE
2 yellow or orange peppers, deseeded
1 large onion, coarsely chopped
400 ml coconut milk
60 g green beans
100 g baby spinach
60 g snow peas

NEARLY NEUTRAL
2 tbsp tamarind liquid
2 tbsp olive oil
$\frac{1}{2}$ cup chicken stock
1 cup bean sprouts

ACID
4 pieces of cod or other firm white fish
1 cup frozen peas

Blend together the peppers, onion, garlic, ginger and chilli.
Pour 2 tablespoons boiling water over 1 tablespoon tamarind
paste and leave it to soak, then strain, reserving the liquid.
Prepare a pan of gently simmering water to poach the cod.
Heat the olive oil, add the pepper paste, lemon grass, lime
leaves and turmeric powder, and stir-fry for another 2–3
minutes. Add the coconut milk and continue to stir-fry for 2–3
minutes. Add the stock and green beans and simmer for 3–4
minutes. Add the cod to the simmering water and poach for
about 5 minutes. Add the peas to the curry sauce and continue
to simmer for another 1–2 minutes, then add the spinach,
snow peas, bean sprouts and tamarind water and cook for
another minute or until the spinach is just wilted. Place a piece
of cod on each plate, spoon over the vegetable curry and

garnish with coriander. Serve with steamed rice, some extra
steamed bok choy or other vegetable dish.

TOMATO, FENNEL AND SEAFOOD STEW
PREPARATION TIME: 5 minutes
COOKING TIME: 20 minutes

HERBS AND SPICES
5–6 garlic cloves, chopped
Black pepper
2 tbsp dill, chopped

ALKALINE
1 medium red onion, coarsely chopped
1 medium fennel, coarsely chopped
400 g vine-ripened tomatoes, roughly chopped

NEARLY NEUTRAL
2–3 tbsp olive oil
1 tbsp tomato paste
1 l vegetable or chicken stock

ACID
125 g green prawns, peeled
125 g small scallops
4 baby squid, cut into rings

Heat the olive oil and sauté the onion and fennel for 3–4
minutes then add the garlic and sauté for another minute.
Add the tomato paste and tomatoes, stir to coat them well
with the oil and sauté for 1–2 minutes. Add the stock and
simmer gently for about 10–15 minutes until the fennel is
soft, then purée. Reheat the soup to a gentle simmer, add the
prawns and squid tentacles and cook for about 1–2 minutes
until the prawns have just turned pink, then add the scallops
and squid rings and continue to cook for another 1–2
minutes. Season with black pepper and serve garnished with
the chopped dill.

NOTE We use fresh uncooked seafood. If you want to use a precooked seafood mixture, add it to the soup at the end of cooking and heat through for a minute at most, or it will be tough and rubbery.

POULTRY AND EGGS

All poultry and eggs are acid forming, so serve them with plenty of vegetables and fruit.

CHICKEN TERIYAKI
PREPARATION TIME: 2 minutes plus 2 hours marinating time
COOKING TIME: 15–20 minutes

ALKALINE
1 tbsp dry white wine

NEARLY NEUTRAL
2 tbsp olive oil
1 tbsp mirin

ACID
4 tbsp light soya sauce
4 chicken breasts, skinned

Shake together the olive oil, mirin, white wine and soya sauce, pour over the chicken breasts and leave to marinate for about 2 hours. Gently fry the chicken breasts and marinade, turning occasionally until the chicken is cooked thoroughly (about 15–20 minutes).

TIP These are delicious served with either the asian noodle salad (page 192) or stir-fried beans with ginger (page 257) and roast sweet potato in soya sauce (page 261).

CHICKEN TERIYAKI KEBABS
These quantities make sufficient for 4 large kebabs or 8 small ones.
PREPARATION TIME: 10 minutes

COOKING TIME: 10 minutes

HERBS AND SPICES
4–8 large garlic cloves, peeled (optional)

ALKALINE
8 cherry tomatoes
2 small zucchini, cut into thick slices
8 shallots cut in half or 6 spring onions cut into 2 cm-length pieces
4–8 small mushrooms

NEARLY NEUTRAL
1 tbsp mirin or rice vinegar
1 tbsp brown sugar

ACID
2 chicken breasts, skinned and cut into equal-sized cubes
2 tbsp teriyaki sauce
1 tbsp soya sauce

Loosely thread the chicken, garlic and vegetables on to skewers, alternating chicken and vegetables. Gently warm through the teriyaki sauce, soya sauce, mirin, and sugar in a small saucepan. Brush the kebabs with the teriyaki sauce and grill or barbecue, continuing to brush the kebabs with the sauce until they are cooked.

VARIATION *Use only spring onions instead of all the other vegetables.*

GARLIC CHICKEN CASSEROLE

PREPARATION TIME: 5 minutes
COOKING TIME: 60–70 minutes

HERBS AND SPICES
12–16 garlic cloves, peeled
4 sprigs thyme

12 sage leaves
1 tsp ground black pepper or to taste

ALKALINE
4–6 shallots, halved
12 baby new potatoes, scrubbed
1 tbsp lemon juice

NEARLY NEUTRAL
1–2 tbsp olive oil
½ cup chicken stock

ACID
6–8 chicken thighs, skinned and boned

Preheat the oven to 170°C. Place the chicken thighs, garlic, shallots, potatoes, thyme, sage and black pepper in an ovenproof casserole dish. Pour over the olive oil, lemon juice and stock. Cover and cook in the oven for 40–45 minutes, then remove the lid and cook for another 20–25 minutes (if you use chicken legs and/or thighs with the bone in, the dish will take slightly longer). Serve with steamed or stir-fried broccoli or bok choy.

INDONESIAN-STYLE CHICKEN NOODLES OR LAKSA

The spices and vegetables balance the meal.
PREPARATION TIME: 15 minutes
COOKING TIME: 15 minutes

HERBS AND SPICES
3–4 garlic cloves, crushed
1 tbsp minced ginger
1 tbsp coriander powder
1 tbsp cumin powder
1½ tsp turmeric powder
1½ tsp cayenne pepper
1 stalk lemon grass, cut into 2 cm slices

3–4 lime leaves
$\frac{1}{2}$ cup fresh coriander, chopped

ALKALINE
6 spring onions, sliced
1 lemon, cut into quarters
150 g spinach or rocket
2–4 baby bok choy, cut in half and then into 2 horizontally to
    separate the leaves and stalk
12 snow peas, cut in half
$\frac{1}{2}$ cup coconut milk or cream

NEARLY NEUTRAL
2 tbsp olive oil
$1\frac{1}{2}$ l chicken or vegetable stock
4 asparagus spears, cut into quarters
1 cup bean sprouts

ACID
2 chicken breasts, skinned
250 g thin rice vermicelli noodles
8 pieces of baby corn, cut in half

Gently poach the chicken breasts for about 10 minutes then
drain, cut into thin slices and keep warm. Heat the oil and add
the garlic, ginger, cumin, coriander, turmeric, cayenne pepper,
lemon grass and lime leaves and stir-fry for 1–2 minutes. Add
the stock and lemon and simmer gently for about 10 minutes.
Remove the lemon, lemon grass and lime leaves, add the
coconut milk and simmer gently. Put the rice noodles in a
bowl, pour over boiling water and leave to stand for about 3–5
minutes, then drain and keep warm. Add the asparagus stems,
bok choy stems, and corn to the stock and continue to simmer
for another 2–3 minutes. Add the spring onions, snow peas,
bean sprouts, asparagus tips, bok choy leaves, spinach or
rocket and simmer for another minute or until the
spinach/rocket has just wilted. Divide the rice noodles
between four large soup bowls, place the chicken slices on the

noodles and pour over the soup and vegetables. Serve garnished with coriander.

POTATO AND SPRING ONION FRITTATA WITH MIXED GREEN SALAD
PREPARATION TIME: 5 minutes
COOKING TIME: 25–30 minutes

HERBS AND SPICES
3–4 large cloves garlic, crushed
Black pepper

ALKALINE
3 medium potatoes, peeled
4 large spring onions, finely sliced
90 g baby spinach
Mixed salad leaves
Cherry tomatoes, halved

NEARLY NEUTRAL
¼ cup olive oil

ACID
4 medium eggs

Boil or steam the potatoes until they are cooked (about 20 minutes); drain and leave to cool. Cut into thin slices. Heat the olive oil in a large sauté pan, add the garlic and spring onions and sauté for about 1 minute. Add the sliced potatoes and continue to sauté for another 3 to 4 minutes until the potato slices are warmed through. Add the spinach and stir until just wilted. Lightly beat the eggs, add black pepper to taste, and pour over the potato. Cook gently, until the base of the omelette is firm and slightly brown. Put the omelette under a hot grill and cook until the top of the frittata sets. Serve with a mixed green salad and some baby tomatoes.

ROAST DUCK BREAST WITH BLACK OLIVE AND MANDARIN SALAD
PREPARATION TIME: 10 minutes
COOKING TIME: 15–20 minutes

HERBS AND SPICES
Black pepper

ALKALINE
120 g mixed watercress, rocket and baby spinach salad leaves
1 red onion, thinly sliced
200 g black olives
2 mandarins, peeled and divided into segments
6 marinated artichokes, halved (optional)
1 tbsp lemon juice

NEARLY NEUTRAL
3 tbsp olive oil

ACID
2–3 duck breasts, skinned
1 tbsp balsamic vinegar

Preheat the oven to 200°C. Pour a little of the olive oil over the duck breasts and bake in the oven for about 15–20 minutes or until cooked to your liking, then slice. Shake together the remaining olive oil, lemon juice and balsamic vinegar. Mix together the mixed spinach, rocket and watercress leaves, onion, olives, mandarin segments and artichokes, pour over the dressing and toss to coat well. Divide the salad among the plates and top with the duck slices, season with black pepper. Serve with a baked potato or boiled new potatoes.

ROAST GINGER CHICKEN LEGS
PREPARATION TIME: 5 minutes plus 3 hours marinating time
COOKING TIME: 45 minutes

HERBS AND SPICES
1 tbsp minced ginger

ALKALINE
1 tbsp lemon juice

NEARLY NEUTRAL
1 tbsp mirin

ACID
4 whole chicken legs, skinned
1 tbsp light soya sauce

Preheat the oven to 200°C. Shake together the ginger, lemon juice, mirin and soya sauce to make the marinade. Place the chicken legs in an ovenproof dish, pour over the marinade and leave for at least 3 hours. Roast the chicken in the oven for approximately 45 minutes (or until no blood oozes from the chicken legs if you pierce them with a skewer). Serve with garlic mashed potato (page 257) and grilled vegetables (page 258).

SPICED DUCK BREAST WITH ASIAN VEGETABLES
PREPARATION TIME: 5 minutes plus marinating time
COOKING TIME: 15 minutes

HERBS AND SPICES
3–4 cloves garlic, crushed
1 tbsp ginger, grated
½ tsp coriander powder
½ tsp cumin powder
½ tsp chilli sambal or cayenne pepper
3 star anise
1 stick cinnamon
½ red chilli, sliced
½ cup fresh coriander

ALKALINE
1 tbsp lemon juice
4 baby bok choy, halved, or soft-stemmed broccoli
4 fresh shiitake or chestnut mushrooms, sliced
2 cups baby spinach leaves
4 spring onions, sliced
60 g snow peas

NEARLY NEUTRAL
2 tbsp olive oil
1 cup chicken or vegetable stock
1 cup bean sprouts

ACID
2–3 duck breasts, skinned and sliced
1 tbsp soya sauce

Mix together the olive oil, lemon juice, garlic, ginger, coriander
powder, cumin powder, and chilli sambal or cayenne pepper.
Add the sliced duck breast and stir to coat it well in the spice
mix and leave to marinate for at least 2 hours or preferably
overnight. Heat the stock with the star anise, cinnamon stick
and chilli and simmer for about 10 minutes, then remove the
star anise and cinnamon stick. Add the bok choy and
mushrooms to the stock and simmer for 2 minutes, then add the
spring onions, snow peas, spinach and bean sprouts and simmer
for another minute until the spinach is just wilted. Add the soya
sauce and heat through. Meanwhile in a separate pan sauté the
duck breast and the marinade for about 5 minutes or until
cooked to your liking. Divide the vegetables and stock between 4
bowls, top with the duck breast and serve garnished with fresh
coriander. This is delicious served with steamed rice or noodles.

SPICY CHICKEN WITH MIXED PEPPER TORTILLAS
PREPARATION TIME: 15 minutes plus 30 minutes marinating
time
COOKING TIME: 20 minutes

HERBS AND SPICES
1 tsp paprika
1 tsp cumin powder
1 tsp coriander powder

ALKALINE
1 tsp lemon juice
2 red peppers, seeded and cut into slices
2 green peppers, seeded and cut into slices
1 large onion, sliced
Tomato salsa*
Guacamole**

NEARLY NEUTRAL
2–3 tbsp olive oil
8 tortillas
Non-dairy sour cream†

ACID
2–3 chicken breasts, sliced
2 tsp balsamic vinegar

Mix together the spices, 1 tablespoon of the olive oil, and the
lemon juice. Add the chicken and stir to ensure the slices are
well coated with the spices and leave to marinate for at least 30
minutes. Toss together the peppers and onion slices, pour over
the remaining olive oil and the balsamic vinegar, ensuring the
peppers and onions are well coated. Sauté the peppers in a
frying pan for about 15–20 minutes until soft. In a separate
pan, sauté the chicken pieces in the marinade for about 5–6
minutes until just cooked. While the chicken is cooking,
sprinkle the tortillas with a little water, wrap them in foil and
put them into a preheated 150°C oven for about 5 minutes to
heat through. To serve, place a tortilla on a plate, add some of
the grilled peppers down the centre, then pieces of the
chicken, topped by a little salsa, guacamole and non-dairy sour
cream. Roll up the tortila, folding in one end, and serve.

† *You can now buy non-dairy sour cream in health food shops. If you can't find it use a little hummus (page 213) instead.*

*TOMATO SALSA
PREPARATION TIME: 5 minutes

HERBS AND SPICES
¼ cup freshly chopped coriander, mint or basil leaves (or a mixture)

ALKALINE
3–4 medium tomatoes, chopped
3–4 spring onions, chopped
1 tbsp lemon juice

Mix together the chopped tomatoes, spring onions and herbs and sprinkle with the lemon juice just before serving.

**GUACAMOLE
PREPARATION TIME: 5 minutes

HERBS AND SPICES
2 tbsp chopped coriander
1 tsp chopped fresh red chilli

ALKALINE
2 avocados, peeled and chopped
1½ tbsp lemon or lime juice
3 spring onions, finely chopped

Toss the avocado in the lemon juice, add the spring onions, coriander and chilli, stir gently and serve immediately.

SPICY CHICKEN WITH MIXED PEPPERS
PREPARATION TIME: 10 minutes plus 1 hour marinating time
COOKING TIME: 10–12 minutes

HERBS AND SPICES
4-5 cloves garlic, crushed
1 tbsp fresh ginger, grated
2 tbsp coarse black pepper
1-2 green or red chillies or to taste
1 cup chopped fresh coriander

ALKALINE
1 red onion, sliced
1 red pepper, seeded and sliced
1 green pepper, seeded and sliced

NEARLY NEUTRAL
2-3 tbsp olive oil

ACID
4-6 boned chicken thighs, sliced

Mix together the garlic, ginger, black pepper and olive oil, pour
over the chicken and marinate for at least 1 hour. Heat a wok or
frying pan and add the chicken and marinade and stir-fry for 3-4
minutes until the chicken is just cooked, then remove the
chicken from the pan and keep warm. Add the onion, peppers
and chilli to the pan and sauté for 3-4 minutes. Add a little water,
cover and fry over a medium heat for another 5-6 minutes until
the vegetables are cooked through. Return the chicken to the pan
and heat through. Serve garnished with coriander.

STIR-FRIED CHICKEN AND VEGETABLES
Replace any of the vegetables listed with any of your favourites.
PREPARATION TIME: 10 minutes
COOKING TIME: 10 minutes

HERBS AND SPICES
3-4 garlic cloves, chopped
1 tbsp ginger, grated
1 red chilli, sliced
Fresh coriander

ALKALINE
1 onion, sliced
2 stalks celery, sliced diagonally into 2 cm pieces
1 red pepper, sliced
8 baby mushrooms
220 g water chestnuts, sliced

NEARLY NEUTRAL
2 tbsp olive oil
½ cup chicken stock
2 tsp mirin or Chinese cooking wine
1 tsp oyster sauce
1 cup bean sprouts

ACID
2 whole chicken breasts, skinned and cut into cubes
2 tsp light soya sauce

Heat the oil and stir-fry the chicken until it is cooked through.
Remove from the pan and keep warm. Add the onion to the
pan and stir-fry for 2–3 minutes then add the garlic, ginger
and chilli and continue to stir-fry for another minute. Add the
celery, pepper and mushrooms, stir to coat them in the oil,
then add the chicken stock, cover and cook for another 2–3
minutes. Add the chicken, water chestnuts, bean sprouts,
mirin, soya sauce and oyster sauce and heat through. Serve
sprinkled with coriander.

THAI-STYLE CHICKEN NOODLES
The spices and vegetables balance the acidity of the chicken and
    noodles, so this is a meal in itself.
PREPARATION TIME: 5 minutes
COOKING TIME: 15 minutes

HERBS AND SPICES
4–5 cloves garlic, crushed
1 tbsp grated ginger
2 long green chillies

2–3 lime leaves
1 stalk lemon grass, cut into 2 cm lengths
Fresh coriander or mint

ALKALINE
1 lemon, quartered
200 g choi sum (or bok choy), cut in half and then into 2
    horizontally to separate the leaves and the stalks
6 spring onions, sliced

NEARLY NEUTRAL
3 tbsp olive oil
1 l chicken stock
100 g bean sprouts

ACID
2–3 chicken breasts, skinned
1 tsp blachen (dried shrimp paste)
250 g rice vermicelli noodles
1 packet prawn crackers* for serving

Poach the chicken breasts for about 10 minutes or until they
are just cooked, drain and cut into slices and keep warm. Heat
the olive oil and stir-fry the garlic, ginger, chillies, lemon grass
and lime leaves for about 30 seconds. Add the chicken stock
and lemon quarters and simmer for about 10 minutes, then
remove the lemon grass, lemon quarters and lime leaves. Add
the chicken and choi sum stalks and simmer gently for 2
minutes. Add the bean sprouts, choi sum leaves, and spring
onions and simmer for another minute. Meanwhile pour
boiling water over the rice vermicelli and leave to stand for
3–5 minutes (or according to the instructions on the packet),
then drain. Divide the noodles between 4 serving plates and
add the chicken and vegetables. Serve garnished with chopped
fresh coriander or mint and serve with prawn crackers.

*Check carefully that the prawn crackers do not contain milk solids as
some of the brands sold in the supermarkets do.*

MEATS NOW AND THEN

GRILLED LAMB CHOPS WITH MINTED SPINACH SALAD
PREPARATION TIME: 10 minutes
COOKING TIME: 15 minutes

HERBS AND SPICES
3–4 tbsp chopped fresh mint

ALKALINE
150 g baby spinach leaves
1 avocado, peeled, stoned and sliced
$\frac{1}{4}$ cantaloupe melon, cut into cubes
$\frac{1}{2}$ red pepper sliced
3–4 spring onions, sliced
1 tbsp lemon juice

NEARLY NEUTRAL
2 tbsp olive oil
1 cup bean sprouts

ACID
8 small lamb loin chops
1 tbsp balsamic vinegar

Grill the lamb chops until cooked to your liking (approximately 15 minutes). Mix together all the salad ingredients. Shake together the olive oil, lemon juice, balsamic vinegar and mint, pour over the salad and toss to coat. Divide the salad between 4 plates and top with the grilled lamb chops.

GRILLED LAMB LOIN WITH NIÇOISE SALAD
PREPARATION TIME: 10 minutes
COOKING TIME: 35 minutes

HERBS AND SPICES
$\frac{1}{4}$ cup chopped wide-leaved parsley

247

¼ cup chopped mint

ALKALINE
8–12 baby new potatoes
60 g green beans
16 cherry tomatoes, halved
½ cup black olives
150 g mixed salad leaves
½ cucumber, cut into cubes
1 tbsp lemon juice

NEARLY NEUTRAL
3 tbsp olive oil

ACID
600 g lamb loin

Preheat the oven to 180°C. Boil or steam the potatoes until cooked. Blanch the green beans in boiling water for about 5 minutes then rinse in cold water. Pour 1 tablespoon oil over the lamb loin and bake for about 35 minutes or until cooked to your liking, leave to stand for about 5 minutes then carve into thick slices. Mix together the salad leaves, potatoes, tomatoes, beans, cucumber, olives, parsley and mint. Shake together the remaining olive oil and lemon juice, pour over the salad, and toss. Divide the salad among 4 plates and top with the grilled lamb slices.

MINCED LAMB KEBABS
There are quite a lot of vegetables and spices in these kebabs which balance the acidity of the lamb. Serving with the aubergine and potato curry (page 255) or the zucchini and pea curry (page 267) with a small amount of steamed white rice (page 208) provides a well-balanced meal.
PREPARATION TIME: 10 minutes
COOKING TIME: 10 minutes

HERBS AND SPICES
4–5 garlic cloves, crushed

1 tbsp fresh ginger, grated
1 green chilli, finely chopped
1 tsp ground cumin
1 tsp ground coriander
1 tsp cayenne pepper
1 tsp garam masala
$\frac{1}{2}$ cup chopped fresh coriander

ALKALINE
1 small onion, finely chopped

NEARLY NEUTRAL
2 tbsp soya yoghurt

ACID
500 g minced lamb (it is preferable to mince your own)

Combine all the ingredients in a mixing bowl, adding the
yoghurt in spoonfuls, ensuring the mixture does not become
too moist. Divide the mixture into smallish balls, thread them
on to a skewer and roll to flatten and lengthen the kebab. Grill,
turning frequently for about 15 minutes or until the kebab is
cooked through.

MINCED PORK IN CRISPY LETTUCE LEAVES
PREPARATION TIME: 10 minutes (if mincing your own pork)
COOKING TIME: 5 minutes

HERBS AND SPICES
2–3 cloves garlic, chopped
1 tsp chilli sambal
$\frac{1}{2}$ cup coriander leaves
$\frac{1}{2}$ cup mint leaves

ALKALINE
1 red onion, finely chopped
2 tbsp lime or lemon juice
1 romaine or iceberg lettuce, leaves separated and washed

NEARLY NEUTRAL
1 tbsp peanut oil
1 tbsp sesame oil

ACID
700 g pork loin, minced
1 tbsp soya sauce

Heat the peanut and sesame oils and sauté the garlic, chilli sambal and minced pork for about 5 minutes until the pork is cooked through. Mix together the pork, onion, lime juice, soya sauce, coriander and mint. Serve large lettuce leaves on to plates and fill with pork.

MINCED PORK WITH NOODLES

PREPARATION TIME: 5 minutes
COOKING TIME: 6-8 minutes

HERBS AND SPICES
4-5 garlic cloves, minced
1 tbsp grated ginger
1-2 fresh large green chillies, finely chopped
$\frac{1}{4}$ cup fresh mint, chopped
$\frac{1}{4}$ cup fresh coriander, chopped

ALKALINE
6 spring onions
180 g baby spinach leaves
100 g snow peas

NEARLY NEUTRAL
2 tbsp olive oil
$\frac{1}{4}$ cup water
2 tbsp mirin (optional)
100 g bean sprouts

ACID
250 g fine egg noodles
500 g pork fillet, minced
¼ cup light soya sauce

Cook the noodles in a large saucepan of boiling water
according to the instructions on the packet and then drain.
While the noodles are cooking, heat the olive oil in a wok and
stir-fry the garlic, ginger and chillies for about a minute. Add
the pork and continue to stir-fry, stirring until all the pork has
changed colour. Add the soya sauce, water and mirin and heat
through. Add the spring onions, spinach, snow peas, bean
sprouts and mint, cover and continue to stir-fry until the
spinach is just wilted. Divide the noodles among four dishes,
top with the pork and vegetables. Serve garnished with
coriander.

MOROCCAN LAMB CASSEROLE
PREPARATION TIME: 5 minutes
COOKING TIME: 1¼ –1½ hours

HERBS AND SPICES
8 garlic cloves, sliced
1 tsp cayenne pepper
1 tsp ground cumin
1 tsp ground coriander
½ tsp ground ginger
½ tsp black pepper
½ cup fresh parsley

ALKALINE
2 small onions, chopped
8 dried apricots, halved
⅓ cup raisins

NEARLY NEUTRAL
2–3 tbsp olive oil
water

ACID
500–600 g diced leg of lamb
2 tbsp ground almonds

Preheat the oven to 180°C. In a large casserole dish, heat the olive oil and sauté the onions for 2–3 minutes, then add the lamb, garlic and all the dry spices. Stir well to coat the lamb with the spices and sauté for 3–4 minutes until all the lamb is browned (don't overcrowd the pan, do it in batches if necessary). Add the raisins, apricots and ground almonds and just cover the meat with water. Cover the dish and cook in the oven for 1¼–1½ hours. Serve garnished with parsley. Serve with steamed rice (page 208) and fresh tomato or tomato salsa (page 243).

RABBIT PILAF
PREPARATION TIME: 10 minutes plus 30 minutes marinating
COOKING TIME: 40–45 minutes

HERBS AND SPICES
3–4 cloves garlic, crushed
½ tsp ground coriander
½ tsp ground cumin
¼ tsp ground turmeric
½ tsp cayenne pepper
1 tsp paprika
¼ tsp ground cinnamon
½ tsp coarse black pepper
1 tbsp mint, chopped
1 tbsp coriander, chopped

ALKALINE
1 onion, finely chopped
½ cup raisins
¼ cup dried apricots, chopped
4 medium vine-ripened tomatoes, chopped
1 tbsp lemon juice

NEARLY NEUTRAL
3 tbsp olive oil
2 cups chicken stock

ACID
2 rabbit portions, skinned, boned and cut into 2 cm pieces
1 cup short-grained rice
1 tbsp pinenuts
1 tbsp flaked almonds

Mix together all the dry spices with the lemon juice and 1
tablespoon of the olive oil in a bowl, add the rabbit pieces
and stir well to coat in the spices and leave to marinate for at
least 30 minutes. In a large sauté pan with a lid heat the oil,
add the rabbit and marinade and sauté until it has changed
colour then remove from the pan and keep warm. Add the
onion to the pan and sauté for 3–4 minutes, then add the
garlic and continue to sauté for another minute before
adding the rabbit, chopped tomatoes, raisins, apricots and
rice. Stir to coat everything in the oil, pour over the chicken
stock, bring to the boil and cover and simmer for about 25
minutes. Remove from heat and leave to stand for about 5
minutes, then stir in the coriander and mint. Serve sprinkled
with pine nuts and almonds.

SPICED LAMB LOIN WITH ROAST VEGETABLES
PREPARATION TIME: 10 minutes plus 2 hours marinating time
COOKING TIME: 30–40 minutes

HERBS AND SPICES
2–3 cloves garlic
$\frac{1}{2}$ tsp black pepper
$\frac{1}{2}$ tsp cayenne pepper
$\frac{1}{2}$ tsp cumin powder
$\frac{1}{2}$ tsp coriander powder
$\frac{1}{2}$ cup fresh coriander, chopped
$\frac{1}{2}$ cup torn fresh basil

ALKALINE
½ medium onion, coarsely chopped
4–8 new potatoes, scrubbed
1 medium to large zucchini, cut in half and thickly sliced
    lengthways
4 vine tomatoes cut in half

NEARLY NEUTRAL
4 tbsp olive oil

ACID
400 g lamb loin

Blend together the garlic, black pepper, cayenne pepper, cumin powder, coriander powder, onion and 2 tablespoons of the olive oil in a food processor. Pour the spice mixture over the lamb and leave to marinate for at least two hours and preferably overnight. Preheat the oven to 180°C. Parboil or steam the potatoes until they are just soft (approximately 10 minutes). Drain, cool and slice thickly. Roast the lamb for approximately 30–40 minutes or until it is cooked to your liking. Put the potatoes, zucchini and tomatoes into a baking dish in one layer, drizzle over the olive oil and stir gently to ensure all the vegetable pieces are covered in oil. Put in the oven 15 minutes after the lamb and cook for about 20–25 minutes. Divide the vegetables among 4 plates, cut the lamb into 4 pieces and place on top of the vegetables. Serve garnished with coriander and basil.

SPICY BARBECUED LEG OF LAMB
PREPARATION TIME: 10 minutes plus 2 hours marinating time
COOKING TIME: 30–40 minutes

HERBS AND SPICES
¼ cup Thai red curry paste
4–5 cloves garlic, peeled

ALKALINE
12 tbsp lemon juice

NEARLY NEUTRAL
2 tbsp olive oil

ACID
1 leg of lamb, butterflied
1 tbsp soya sauce

Mix together the curry paste, garlic, lemon juice, olive oil and soya sauce. Make a few jabs in the lamb, pour over the spice mixture and leave to marinate for at least two hours and preferably overnight. Barbecue the lamb for approximately 45–50 minutes or until it is cooked to your liking. Leave to stand for 10 minutes before carving into thick slices. Serve with green beans with ginger (page 257), citrus salsa (page 197) and spicy mashed potatoes (page 264).

VITAL VEGETABLES

TIP *If you have osteoporosis, use potatoes whenever possible to replace cereals such as bread, rice or pasta with meat, egg or fish dishes.*

AUBERGINE AND POTATO CURRY
PREPARATION TIME: 20 minutes plus soaking time
COOKING TIME: 30 minutes

HERBS AND SPICES
4–5 cloves garlic, crushed
1 tbsp grated ginger
2 tsp mustard seeds
2 tsp curry powder
6–8 curry leaves (optional)
1 green chilli
2–3 tbsp chopped fresh coriander

ALKALINE
450 g potatoes
1 medium aubergine (about 300 g)

1 onion, sliced
1 tbsp lemon juice

NEARLY NEUTRAL
2 tbsp olive oil
2 tbsp tamarind paste

Boil the potatoes until cooked, then cool, peel and chop them into cubes. Cut the aubergine into similar-sized cubes. Pour $\frac{1}{2}$ cup of boiling water over 2 tablespoons of tamarind paste and leave to soak for 30 minutes, strain and reserve the liquid. Heat the olive oil and add the mustard seeds. When the mustard seeds begin to pop add the onion and sauté for 3–4 minutes until it changes colour, then add the curry powder, curry leaves, chilli, garlic and ginger and continue to sauté for another 1–2 minutes. Add the aubergine, tamarind liquid and $\frac{1}{2}$ cup of water and simmer for about 15 minutes until the aubergine is almost cooked. Stir in the potatoes and continue to cook until the potatoes and aubergine are cooked through. Sprinkle with the lemon juice and serve garnished with fresh chopped coriander.

BAKED SESAME MUSHROOMS
PREPARATION TIME: 10 minutes
COOKING TIME: 15–20 minutes

HERBS AND SPICES
2 cloves garlic, crushed
1 tbsp chopped parsley

ALKALINE
8–12 large or medium mushrooms, peeled and stems removed
2 tbsp celery, very finely chopped
1 tsp lemon juice

NEARLY NEUTRAL
1 tbsp sesame seeds
2 tbsp tahini
2 tbsp soya yoghurt or soya cream

ACID
1 tbsp tamari or light soya sauce

Preheat the oven to 200°C. Mix together all the ingredients except the mushrooms. Top each mushroom with some of the filling and bake in the oven for 15–20 minutes

GARLIC MASHED POTATOES
PREPARATION TIME: 5 minutes
COOKING TIME: 20–25 minutes

HERBS AND SPICES
3–4 garlic cloves, crushed
chopped fresh parsley

ALKALINE
4–5 potatoes
2 tbsp lemon juice

NEARLY NEUTRAL
2–3 tbsp olive oil

Boil or steam the unpeeled potatoes until tender, then drain, cool slightly and peel. Mash together the garlic and potatoes and slowly add the olive oil and the lemon juice, continuing mashing until the potato forms a thick smooth paste. Serve sprinkled with parsley.

VARIATION *Roast a whole garlic in the oven, then peel the cloves and mash with the potato.*

GREEN BEANS WITH GINGER
PREPARATION TIME: 2 minutes
COOKING TIME: 7–8 minutes

HERBS AND SPICES
1 tbsp fresh ginger, grated
½ tsp chilli sambal

ALKALINE
450 g green beans, topped and tailed

NEARLY NEUTRAL
2 tbsp olive oil

Heat the olive oil, add the beans and sauté for about 3–4 minutes. Add the ginger and chilli sambal and continue to sauté for another 2–3 minutes or until the beans are cooked but still crisp.

GRILLED VEGETABLES

Choose any selection of your favourite vegetables to make a delicious, healthy starter or to accompany grilled or baked fish or meat.

PREPARATION TIME: 10 minutes
COOKING TIME: 5–10 minutes if grilling or 30 minutes if roasting

HERBS AND SPICES
8–12 cloves garlic, peeled (optional)

ALKALINE
$\frac{1}{2}$ red pepper, seeded and cut into 4 pieces
$\frac{1}{2}$ green pepper, seeded and cut into 4 pieces
4 large field mushrooms
1 small fennel bulb, cut horizontally into slices
4 vine tomatoes, halved
2 chicory heads, cut in half

NEARLY NEUTRAL
4 pieces asparagus cut into $2\frac{1}{2}$ cm lengths
2–3 tbsp olive oil

ACID
1 small fresh corn cob cut into 4, or 12–16 baby corn pieces

Toss all the vegetables in the olive oil and grill or roast until they are cooked. Grilling makes them crisper than roasting and takes much less time. If vegetables are roasted, it is better to cook the mushrooms in a separate pan.

MASHED PARSNIP POTATOES
PREPARATION TIME: 2–3 minutes
COOKING TIME: 20–25 minutes

HERBS AND SPICES
1 tsp cumin powder
Black pepper to taste
Chopped fresh parsley

ALKALINE
3 large potatoes, scrubbed and cut into large pieces
3 small parsnips, peeled and cut into large chunks

NEARLY NEUTRAL
2–3 tbsp olive oil
$\frac{1}{3}$ cup soya cream or milk

Boil or steam the potatoes and parsnips in separate pans until they are cooked. Mash all the ingredients together to form a smooth thick paste, add the soya cream or milk slowly to get the right consistency. Season with black pepper and serve sprinkled with parsley.

POACHED LEEKS WITH LEMON DRESSING
This recipe was given to us by Chris Williams.
PREPARATION TIME: 2 minutes
COOKING TIME: 15–20 minutes

HERBS AND SPICES
$\frac{1}{2}$ bunch of fresh wide-leaved parsley
1 tsp black pepper

ALKALINE
5–6 leeks, white part only, cleaned and cut in half lengthways
2 tsp lemon zest
1 tbsp fresh lemon juice

NEARLY NEUTRAL
5 tbsp olive oil

In a large pan, bring enough water to cover the leeks to a
gentle simmer, then add the leeks and cook for about 15–20
minutes until they are tender. Purée the parsley, lemon zest,
olive oil and pepper in a food processor. Arrange the leeks on a
serving dish, drizzle over the parsley mixture, sprinkle with
lemon juice and freshly ground black pepper to taste. This dish
can be served hot or cold, garnished with extra parsley.

POTATO AND PEA CURRY
PREPARATION TIME: 5–10 minutes
COOKING TIME: 20–25 minutes

HERBS AND SPICES
3–4 garlic cloves, crushed
1 tsp fresh ginger, grated
1 tsp cumin seeds
1 tsp turmeric
1 red chilli, chopped
1 tsp garam masala
$\frac{1}{2}$ cup chopped fresh coriander

ALKALINE
1 large onion, sliced
250 g potatoes, washed and scrubbed
1 tbsp lemon juice

NEARLY NEUTRAL
3 tbsp olive oil
$\frac{1}{2}$ cup water

ACID
2 cups fresh peas

Parboil or steam the potatoes, then cut them into cubes. Heat
the olive oil and stir-fry the onion for 3–4 minutes, then add

the garlic, ginger, cumin seeds, turmeric and chilli and continue to stir-fry for another minute. Add the potatoes and fresh peas and stir to coat them with the spices. Add the water and cook for about 10–15 minutes until the potatoes are soft, add lemon juice and continue to cook for another 5 minutes adding a little more water as necessary. Serve sprinkled with garam masala and coriander.

NOTE *If using frozen peas add them with the lemon juice.*
VARIATION *Add baby mushrooms and/or corn.*

ROAST SWEET POTATOES WITH SOYA SAUCE
PREPARATION TIME: 5 minutes
COOKING TIME: 30 minutes

HERBS AND SPICES
1 tsp grated nutmeg

ALKALINE
3–4 medium sweet potatoes, peeled and cut into thick slices

NEARLY NEUTRAL
1–2 tbsp olive oil
2 tbsp light soya sauce

Preheat the oven to 200°C. Pour the olive oil in to a roasting tin, add the potatoes and toss to coat them in the oil. Pour over the soya sauce and sprinkle with grated nutmeg. Bake in the oven for about 30 minutes or until the potatoes are just cooked.

SAUTÉED BOK CHOY WITH WORCESTER SAUCE
Worcester sauce is a good substitute for tamarind liquid and also for soya sauce.
PREPARATION TIME: 1 minute
COOKING TIME: 3–4 minutes

HERBS AND SPICES
3-4 cloves garlic, chopped

ALKALINE
4-8 baby bok choy, cut in half and then into 2 horizontally to separate the leaves and stalks

NEARLY NEUTRAL
1 tbsp olive oil
1 tbsp Worcester sauce
2 tbsp water

Heat the olive oil and briefly stir-fry the garlic. Add the bok choy stalks, stir to coat in the oil, add the Worcester sauce and water, cover and cook for 1-2 minutes. Add the bok choy leaves and continue to cook for another minute.

SAUTÉED CAULIFLOWER WITH TOMATOES AND CAPERS
PREPARATION TIME: 5-6 minutes
COOKING TIME: 30 minutes

HERBS AND SPICES
2-3 cloves garlic, crushed
1 red chilli (or to taste), chopped
1 cup fresh coriander or parsley, chopped Black pepper

ALKALINE
1 small or medium cauliflower, cut into florets
12-16 cherry tomatoes
5-6 spring onions, sliced
2-3 heaped tbsp small capers

NEARLY NEUTRAL
2-3 tbsp olive oil

Steam or boil the cauliflower until cooked. Heat the olive oil in a wok, add the garlic, chilli and capers and sauté for 1-2 minutes. Add the cooked cauliflower and tomatoes and sauté until the tomatoes are just cooked through with their skins beginning to burst. Add the spring onions, season with black pepper to taste and continue to sauté for another minute. Stir through the coriander or parsley and serve immediately. This is delicious served by itself as a main course or with grilled or baked fish or meat.

SAUTÉED SWEET POTATO WITH RAISINS AND PINE NUTS
PREPARATION TIME: 5 minutes
COOKING TIME: 30 minutes

HERBS AND SPICES
2–3 cloves garlic, crushed
1 tsp ground cinnamon
1 tsp black pepper

ALKALINE
1 onion, sliced
500 g sweet potato, peeled and cut into cubes
3 tbsp raisins

NEARLY NEUTRAL
3 tbsp olive oil
2 tbsp water

ACID
3 tbsp pine nuts

Heat the olive oil and sauté the onion for 3–4 minutes, add the garlic and continue to stir-fry for another minute. Add the sweet potato and continue to sauté for 5 minutes, tossing so that it is coated in the olive oil. Add the raisins, black pepper, cinnamon and water, cover and simmer for about 20 minutes, stirring occasionally until the potato is soft. Dry fry the pine nuts until they start to turn colour and sprinkle over the sweet potato.

SPICY MASHED POTATOES
PREPARATION TIME: 5 minutes
COOKING TIME: 25 minutes

HERBS AND SPICES
½ tsp mustard seeds
4–5 garlic cloves, crushed
1 green chilli, chopped
½ tsp turmeric powder
½ tsp cumin powder
½ tsp coriander powder
½ tsp cayenne pepper
2–3 tbsp chopped mint

ALKALINE
500 g potatoes
1 tbsp fresh lemon juice
1 onion, chopped

NEARLY NEUTRAL
4 tbsp olive oil

Boil the potatoes for about 20 minutes in a large pan until they are cooked, then peel and mash them with the lemon juice and 2 tablespoons of the olive oil. Heat the remaining olive oil in a frying pan and fry the mustard seeds until they begin to pop, add the onion and sauté for 3–4 minutes. Add the garlic, chilli and dry spices and continue to fry for another minute, then mix them into the potato with the mint.

STIR-FRIED FENNEL AND POTATO
PREPARATION TIME: 5 minutes
COOKING TIME: 20 minutes

HERBS AND SPICES
3–4 cloves garlic, chopped
½ cup chopped fresh parsley

ALKALINE
3-4 medium potatoes
1 fennel bulb, diced
1 onion, chopped

NEARLY NEUTRAL
3-4 tbsp olive oil

Parboil or steam the potatoes for about 10 minutes then cool
slightly and cut them into cubes. Sauté the onion in the olive
oil for 2-3 minutes then add the garlic, potato and fennel and
stir-fry over a moderate heat until the potato is crispy. Stir
through the parsley and serve immediately.

STIR-FRIED SPINACH AND BEAN SPROUTS
PREPARATION TIME: 1 minute
COOKING TIME: 2-3 minutes

HERBS AND SPICES
2-3 cloves garlic, crushed

ALKALINE
180 g baby spinach leaves
6 spring onions, sliced

NEARLY NEUTRAL
2 tbsp olive oil
100 g bean sprouts

ACID
1 tbsp soya sauce

Wash the spinach and shake, but leave excess water clinging to
the leaves. Heat the olive oil and briefly sauté the garlic and
spring onions for about a minute. Add the spinach, bean
sprouts and soya sauce and continue to sauté for another
minute or until the spinach has just wilted.

STUFFED GREEN PEPPERS
PREPARATION TIME: 10 minutes
COOKING TIME: 45 minutes

HERBS AND SPICES
1 red chilli, finely chopped
½ cup fresh mint or parsley, finely chopped

ALKALINE
4 large green peppers, halved and seeded
1 small onion, finely chopped
2 sticks of celery, finely chopped
2 vine-ripened tomatoes, finely chopped
4 medium carrots, juiced

NEARLY NEUTRAL
2 cups water
2–3 tbsp olive oil

ACID
1 cup basmati rice
½ cup frozen peas
½ cup frozen corn

Cook the rice according to the instructions on (page 208).
Brush the peppers generously with some of the olive oil. Mix
together all the remaining ingredients, including the remaining
oil and fill each pepper with the mixture. Bake in a preheated
200°C oven for 30 minutes.

VEGETABLE CURRY
PREPARATION TIME: 5 minutes
COOKING TIME: 20–25 minutes

HERBS AND SPICES
2–3 garlic cloves, chopped
1 tsp fresh ginger, grated
1 green chilli, chopped

1½ tsp garam masala
½ tsp turmeric
½ tsp cayenne pepper
½ cup fresh coriander, chopped

ALKALINE
500 g baby new potatoes
1 onion, sliced
200 g baby mushrooms
6 medium vine-ripened tomatoes, sliced

NEARLY NEUTRAL
3 tbsp olive oil
½ cup water

ACID
1 cup fresh or frozen peas
1 cup fresh or frozen corn
½ cup soya yoghurt or coconut cream

Parboil the potatoes for 15 minutes, then drain. Heat the olive oil and stir-fry the onion for 2–3 minutes, then add the garlic, ginger, chilli, garam masala, turmeric and cayenne pepper and continue to stir-fry for another minute. Add the potatoes, mushrooms, tomatoes, peas, corn and water, cover and simmer for about 10 minutes (if using frozen peas add after about 8 minutes and continue to cook until they are heated through). Stir through the soya yoghurt or coconut cream and heat through. Serve garnished with the coriander.

ZUCCHINI AND PEA CURRY
PREPARATION TIME: 5 minutes
COOKING TIME: 10 minutes

HERBS AND SPICES
3–4 garlic cloves, crushed
1 tbsp fresh ginger, grated
1 tsp cumin powder

½ tsp turmeric powder
1 tsp chilli sambal or ½ tsp cayenne pepper
½ cup chopped fresh coriander

ALKALINE
1 onion, chopped
300 g zucchini, sliced
1 cup fresh peas
4–6 spring onions, sliced

NEARLY NEUTRAL
2 tbsp olive oil
½ cup water

Heat the olive oil and stir-fry the onion for 2–3 minutes, then add the garlic, ginger, cumin, turmeric and chilli sambal and stir-fry for another minute. Add the zucchini, spring onions and peas and stir to coat in the spices. Add the water, cover and simmer gently for about 5 minutes until the zucchini is soft. Serve sprinkled with the chopped coriander.

DELICIOUS DESSERTS

The best dessert is a plate of fresh fruit. However, here are some simple and delicious alternatives.

TIP If you don't have an ice-cream maker, you can make a sorbet, or even soya ice cream as follows: freeze the mixture until it is almost set, then remove it from the freezer and stir well to break up the ice crystals. Finally, return the mixture to the freezer until it sets.

BAKED PLUMS WITH MACAROONS
PREPARATION TIME: 5 minutes
COOKING TIME: 20–25 minutes

ALKALINE
6 large plums, halved and stoned

NEARLY NEUTRAL
⅓ cup kirsch or Amaretto

ACID
75 g macaroons, crushed

Preheat the oven to 180°C. Put the crushed macaroons in the bottom of a small baking dish. Put the plums on top of the macaroons, sprinkle with kirsch and bake for about 20 minutes or until the plums are well cooked through and soft.

CHILLED WATERMELON DESSERT
PREPARATION TIME: 10 minutes plus chilling time
COOKING TIME: 5 minutes

ALKALINE
600 g watermelon flesh
Juice of half a lemon

NEARLY NEUTRAL
30 g caster sugar
Soya cream to serve
2 tbsp ginger wine or vodka (optional)

ACID
1 tbsp cornflour

Purée the watermelon in a food processor and push through a coarse sieve to remove any remaining seeds. Put the watermelon and caster sugar in a saucepan and bring to a slow simmer, stirring to dissolve the sugar. Mix the cornflour with just enough water to form a smooth paste, then pour it into the watermelon syrup. Stir continuously until the watermelon begins to boil and thicken, and continue to cook for 2 minutes. Add the lemon juice, stir and allow to cool slightly. Transfer into serving dishes and chill in the fridge. Serve with soya cream with a little ginger wine or vodka poured over it.

VARIATION *Make watermelon jelly using agar-agar and eliminating the cornflour.*

EGG CUSTARD WITH BERRIES
PREPARATION TIME: 5 minutes
COOKING TIME: 5 minutes

ALKALINE
1 punnet fresh raspberries
1 punnet fresh blueberries

NEARLY NEUTRAL
$\frac{1}{2}$ cup raw cane caster sugar
4 tbsp soya cream
$1\frac{1}{2}$ tbsp Grand Marnier or Drambuie

ACID
4 egg yolks

Beat the egg yolks and sugar with a little water in a heatproof bowl until the mixture becomes pale yellow in colour. Heat the mixture gently over a saucepan of boiling water and continue to whisk until it thickens and coats the back of a wooden spoon. Remove from the heat and continue to whisk for a few minutes until the mixture cools, stir in the soya cream and Grand Marnier or Drambuie, cover and leave to cool. Divide the fruit between four dishes and pour over the custard.

GINGER KIWIFRUIT SORBET
PREPARATION TIME: 5 minutes plus chilling time
COOKING TIME: 10 minutes

HERBS AND SPICES
$\frac{1}{2}$ tsp grated preserved ginger

ALKALINE
4 kiwi fruit, peeled
1 tbsp lime juice

NEARLY NEUTRAL
$^1/_3$ cup raw cane sugar
1 cup water
$^1/_4$ cup ginger wine

Combine the sugar, water and ginger wine in a pan, stir until
the sugar is dissolved, and gently boil for about 5 minutes.
Purée the kiwifruit and preserved ginger with the syrup and
lime juice. Chill in the fridge and then process in an ice-cream
maker.

MANDARIN AND CAMPARI SORBET WITH BLUEBERRIES
PREPARATION TIME: 5 minutes plus freezing
COOKING TIME: 5 minutes

ALKALINE
1 cup freshly squeezed mandarin juice (about 5 mandarins)
Juice of one small lemon
200 g blueberries

NEARLY NEUTRAL
$^1/_2$ cup raw cane sugar
$^1/_2$ cup water
$^1/_4$ cup Campari (optional)

Dissolve the sugar in the water and simmer briskly for 4–5
minutes to make a syrup then leave to cool. Mix the mandarin
and lemon juice, sugar syrup and Campari together and put
into the fridge to cool. Process in an ice-cream maker. Serve
with fresh blueberries.

MINTED ORANGES IN RED WINE
PREPARATION TIME: 10 minutes plus cooling time
COOKING TIME: 15 minutes

HERBS AND SPICES
1 cinnamon stick

4 cloves
2-3 tbsp fresh mint, finely chopped

ALKALINE
4 oranges, peeled and sectioned
1 tbsp lemon juice
1 tbsp lemon peel

NEARLY NEUTRAL
¼ cup sugar
½ cup water
½ cup red wine or Campari

Gently simmer the sugar, water, red wine or Campari, cinnamon, cloves, and lemon juice for about 15 minutes, then strain. Put the oranges in a serving dish, pour over the syrup, sprinkle with the mint and leave to cool.

POACHED RED GRAPES
PREPARATION TIME: 1-2 minutes
COOKING TIME: 10 minutes

HERBS AND SPICES
1 cinnamon stick

ALKALINE
400 g red grapes, washed and dried
125 g raisins
1 cup grape juice or red wine
1 tbsp lemon juice

NEARLY NEUTRAL
½ cup organic unrefined caster sugar

Combine grape juice or red wine, sugar, raisins and cinnamon and simmer briskly for 5 minutes. Add the grapes and continue to simmer for another 5 minutes. Add the lemon juice. Serve with soya cream.

RASPBERRY ZABAGLIONE

PREPARATION TIME: 15 minutes plus cooling time
COOKING TIME: 5–7 minutes

ALKALINE
2 punnets raspberries or 500 g packet of frozen raspberries

NEARLY NEUTRAL
$^1\!/_2$ cup sweet sherry
1 tsp icing sugar or to taste
$^1\!/_2$ cup raw caster sugar
$^1\!/_2$ cup soya cream
2 tbsp Cointreau
1 cup extra soya cream to serve

ACID
'Savoiardi' biscuits
4 large egg yolks

Cover the bottom of a glass serving bowl with the Savoiardi
biscuits, and add one punnet of raspberries. Pour over the
sherry and gently shake the bowl to make sure all the biscuits
are covered. Purée the other punnet of raspberries with the
icing sugar and pour over the layer of raspberries. Put the eggs,
caster sugar and a little water into a heatproof bowl and beat
together until the mixture turns pale yellow and creamy.
Gently heat the egg mixture over a saucepan of boiling water,
whisking continuously for about 5 minutes until the mixture
doubles in volume and becomes thick and forms soft peaks (do
not let the mixture boil or the eggs will curdle). Stir in the soya
cream and Cointreau then pour the zabaglione over the
raspberries and put in the fridge to cool. Serve with additional
soya cream.

RED GRAPEFRUIT AND GIN SORBET

PREPARATION TIME: 5 minutes plus freezing
COOKING TIME: 5 minutes

ALKALINE
1 cup freshly squeezed red grapefruit juice (about 2 grapefruits)
Juice of one small lemon
200 g blueberries

NEARLY NEUTRAL
$\frac{1}{2}$ cup raw cane sugar
$\frac{1}{2}$ cup water
$\frac{1}{3}$ cup gin (optional)

Dissolve the sugar in the water over a low heat, and simmer for 4–5 minutes to make a syrup and leave to cool. Mix together the grapefruit and lemon juice, sugar syrup and gin and put into the fridge to cool. Process in an ice-cream maker. Serve with fresh blueberries.

RUM AND RAISIN COCONUT CRÈME CARAMELS (makes 8 individual ramekins)
PREPARATION TIME: 10 minutes plus marinating time
COOKING TIME: 60 minutes

ALKALINE
$\frac{1}{2}$ cup raisins
1 cup coconut milk
$\frac{1}{2}$ cup coconut cream

NEARLY NEUTRAL
$\frac{1}{2}$ cup molasses
$\frac{1}{2}$ cup water
2 tbsp dark rum
$\frac{1}{4}$ cup caster sugar

ACID
3 medium eggs
1 egg yolk

Put the molasses and water in a saucepan, bring to a gentle boil, stirring to dissolve the sugar, then leave to boil for about 5 minutes. Remove from the heat, stir in the rum and add about a dessertspoon full of the syrup to each ramekin. Pour the remaining syrup over the raisins and leave to marinate for at least 4 hours or overnight if possible. Preheat the oven to 160°C. Whisk together the eggs and sugar, then whisk in the coconut milk and coconut cream and divide among the ramekins. Put the ramekins into a baking tray with enough water to come halfway up the sides of the ramekins and bake them in the oven for 45–50 minutes. Remove from the oven, allow to cool and refrigerate. Tip the crèmes upside down on to serving plates and serve with the raisins and extra syrup.

STRAWBERRIES WITH PINE NUTS
PREPARATION TIME: 5 minutes

ALKALINE
400 g strawberries

NEARLY NEUTRAL
1 tbsp sugar
Coconut or soya cream

ACID
¼ cup pine nuts

Purée half the strawberries with the sugar and pine nuts. Slice the remaining strawberries, divide among four plates and pour over the strawberry and pine nut purée. Serve with coconut or soya cream.

TOFU ICE-CREAM
PREPARATION TIME: 5 minutes plus freezing time

ALKALINE
1 cup fresh orange juice
450 g ripe bananas, peeled and sliced

NEARLY NEUTRAL
2 tbsp honey

ACID
150 g soft tofu

Purée all the ingredients together in a food processor. Put in the freezer for about 4 hours until frozen but not solid.

CAKES

APRICOT AND PECAN RUM TORTE
PREPARATION TIME: 10 minutes plus chilling time
COOKING TIME: 50 minutes

ALKALINE
175 g dried apricots
175 g raisins

NEARLY NEUTRAL
125 g dark muscovado sugar
2 tbsp dark rum
$\frac{1}{2}$ tsp salt

ACID
120 g pecan nuts
7 egg whites
4 tsp cornflour

Preheat the oven to 160°C. Coarsely chop or process the apricots and nuts and mix with the raisins, cornflour and rum. Beat the egg whites with the salt until they form soft peaks then slowly add the sugar, continuously beating until the mixture forms stiff peaks. Fold the fruit mix into the egg whites then pour into a greased or lined 24 cm springform cake tin and bake for 50 minutes. Allow the cake to cool in the oven with the door open. Refrigerate for at least 4 hours before serving. Serve cold with soya cream and some fresh berries.

VARIATION Use dried dates, figs or prunes instead of the raisins, or use walnuts or almonds instead of the pecans.

MIXED FRUIT, FAT-FREE CAKE

This recipe was given to us by Robin Pavett.
PREPARATION TIME: 10 minutes plus overnight soaking
COOKING TIME: 1–1 ½ hours

ALKALINE
450 g mixed fruit
1 tbsp lemon juice
1 tsp lemon rind

NEARLY NEUTRAL
1 cup dark muscovado sugar
200 ml cold tea

ACID
1 small egg
1 cup self-raising flour

Soak the dried fruit and sugar in the tea overnight. Preheat the oven to 180°C. Add the egg, flour, lemon rind and juice to the fruit and mix well. Put into a loaf tin and bake for about 1–1½ hours.

PEAR AND KIWIFRUIT CAKE

PREPARATION TIME: 15 minutes
COOKING TIME: 50–55 minutes

ALKALINE
3 kiwifruit, peeled and sliced
500 g fresh brown skinned pears (Conference), peeled, sliced lengthways and cored
1 tbsp lemon juice

NEARLY NEUTRAL
¼ cup soya milk

1 tsp grapeseed oil
½ tsp salt

ACID
2 medium eggs
1½ cups flour
½ cup cane sugar
½ cup sliced almonds

Heat the oven to 190°C and grease a cake tin with the grapeseed oil and sprinkle over the chopped almonds. Shake the pan to distribute the almonds across the base. Prepare the fruit and toss in lemon juice to prevent discolouring. Beat together the eggs and soya milk until they become pale yellow in colour then add the sugar and continue to beat until the mixture forms ribbons. Gently fold in the flour and salt, and then add the pears and kiwifruit and stir to mix well. Pour the cake mix into the cake tin and bake for about 50–55 minutes. This cake is very moist and is best eaten straight away.

GLOSSARY

Aubergine Also known as eggplant.

Bamboo shoots Sold canned in water. Once removed from the can, they will keep in the fridge, covered by cold water which should be changed daily.

Bean sprouts Shoots of mung beans or soya beans. These can now be bought fresh in most supermarkets. Fresh bean sprouts will keep for up to a week in the fridge, if covered by water, changed regularly. They are available canned and should be rinsed before use.

Blacan Dried shrimp paste.

Bok choy A variety of Chinese cabbage, now commonly available in supermarkets and all Asian food shops.

Chicory Also known as Belgian endive or wikhof.

Chillies Fresh chillies can be stored in the freezer. The seeds are the hottest part and can be removed if you like a milder taste.

Chinese rice wine Dry sherry can be substituted.

Choy sum Flowering Chinese cabbage.

Coriander Also known as cilantro.

Dashi A basic stock made from dried bonito flakes and kombu (seaweed) used in Japanese cooking.

Dried shiitake mushrooms Have a unique flavour, need to be soaked in hot water to rehydrate them.

Fish sauce Oyster sauce could be substituted.

Kiwi fruit Also known as Chinese gooseberry.

Lemon grass Substitute lemon peel or a whole lemon cut into quarters.

Mirin A sweet low-alcohol rice wine. Can be substituted by a medium or sweet sherry or white vermouth or Chinese cooking wine.

Miso A thick salty paste made with fermented soya beans, barley or other cereals. It is very high in protein and can be used in sauces and soups. Miso varies in colour from light creamy yellow to dark red brown, the darker-coloured varieties tending to be more salty.

Nori Sheets of dried, paper-thin seaweed. It should be crisped over a low flame before use in sushi or in salads.

Rocket Also known as arugula.

Sesame oil Made from roasted, crushed white sesame seeds, use for flavouring rather than cooking.

Snow peas Also known as mangetout.

Soya sauce There are many varieties, including light soya sauce. The Japanese shoyu or tamari are best in salad dressings.

Spring onions Also known as scallions, occasionally as shallots (not to be confused with the small red or brown onions called shallots).

Sweet potato Also known as kumara.

Tamarind Usually found semi-dried. Mix with hot water, leave to stand for ten to fifteen minutes, then strain. It can be found in some Asian shops as a concentrated paste which is used as it is. Worcestershire sauce could be used as a substitute.

Zucchini Also known as courgette.

NOTES

Introduction

1 Plant, Jane, 2001. *Your Life in Your Hands*. Paperback edition. Virgin Books.

2 Plant, Jane and Tidey, Gill, 2002. *The Plant Programme*. Paperback edition. Virgin Books.

3 National Osteoporosis Society Online. http://www.nos.org.uk/osteo.asp

4 http://www.osteoporosis.ca/OSTEO/D01-01.html

5 Campbell, T. C. and Junshi, C., 1994. Diet and chronic degenerative disease perspectives from China. *American Journal of Clinical Nutrition*, 59, Supplement, 11, 535–11, 615.

6 Author unknown. Quoted in Petty, Mike (editor), 2001. *Eden Project: The Guide*. Eden Project Books.

Chapter 1: Bones of Contention

1 http://www.osteo.org (the National Institutes of Health Osteoporosis and Related Bone Diseases – National Resource Centre, USA)

2 http://www.osteoporosis.ca (the Osteoporosis Society of Canada)

3 http://www.nos.org.uk (the National Osteoporosis Society in the UK)

4 Plant, Jane, 2001. *Your Life in Your Hands*. Paperback edition. Virgin Books.

5 Plant, Jane and Tidey, Gill, 2002. *The Plant Programme*. Paperback edition. Virgin Books.

6 http://www.nof.org/news/pressreleases/prevmo_2001.html

7 http://www.osteo.org (the National Institutes of Health Osteoporosis and Related Bone Diseases – National Resource Centre, USA)

8 http://www.osteoporosis.ca (the Osteoporosis Society of Canada)

9 http://www.nos.org.uk (the National Osteoporosis Society in the UK)

10 Riis, B. J., 1993. Biochemical markers of bone turnover. II. Diagnosis, prophylaxis, and treatment of osteoporosis. *American Journal of Medicine*, 95(5A), 17–21S.

11 Assessment of fracture risk and its application to screening for post-menopausal osteoporosis: report of a WHO Study Group. *World Health Organisation Technical Report*, Series 843, 1994, 1–129.

12 Johnston, C. C. Jr and Melton J. L. 3rd, 1995. Bone densitometry. In: Riggs, B. L. and Melton, L. J. 3rd, editors. *Osteoporosis: etiology, diagnosis, and management*. Second edition. Philadelphia: Lippincott-Raven, 275–297.

13 Lee, J. R., 1999. *Natural Progesterone*. Second revised edition. Jon Carpenter.

14 http://www.osteo.org/osteo.html

15 http://www.osteoporosis.ca

16 http://www.nos.org.uk

17 http://www.postgradmed.com/issues/1998/10_98/goddard.htm

18 Greenspan, S. L., Myers, E. R., Maitland, L. A. and others, 1994. Fall severity and bone mineral density as risk factors for hip fracture in ambulatory elderly. *Journal of the American Medical Association*, 271 (2), 128–133.

19 Hemenway, D., Feskanich, D. and Colditz, G. A. 1995. Body height and hip fracture: a cohort study of 90,000 women. *International Journal of Epidemiology*, 24 (4), 783–786.

20 Hemenway, D., Azrael, D. R., Rimm, E. B. and others, 1994. Risk factors for hip fracture in US men aged 40 through 75 years. *American Journal of Public Health*, 84 (11), 1843–1845.

21 Cummings, S. R., Nevitt, M. C., Browner, W. S. and others, 1995. Risk factors for hip fracture in white women: Study of Osteoporotic Fractures Research Group. *New England Journal of Medicine*, 332 (12), 767–773.

22 http://www.who.int/nut/malnutrition_worldwide.html

23 Bootsma, G. P., Dekhuijzen, P. N., Festen, J. and others, 1997. Effects of inhaled corticosteroids on bone. *Netherlands Journal of Medicine*, 50 (6), 254–260.

24 Lonning, P. E. 1998. Aromatase inhibitors and their future role in post-menopausal women with early breast cancer. *British Journal of Cancer*, 78, suppl 4, 12–15.

25 Wysowski, D. K., Baum, C., Ferguson, W. J. and others, 1996. Sedative-hypnotic drugs and the risk of hip fracture. *Journal of Clinical Epidemiology*, 49 (1), 111–113.

26 Cromer, B. A., Blair, J. M. Mahan, J. D. and others, 1996. A prospective comparison of bone density in adolescent girls receiving depot medroxy-progesterone acetate (Depo-Provera), levonorgestrel (Norplant), or oral contraceptives. *Journal of Pediatrics*, 129 (5), 671–676.

27 Lee, John R., 1999. *Natural Progesterone*. Second revised edition. Jon Carpenter.

28 e.g. http://www.osteo.org/

29 Plant, Jane, 2001. *Your Life in Your Hands*. Paperback edition. Virgin Books.

30 Personal communication to Jane Plant.

31 Peto, R. and others, 2000. Smoking, smoking cessation and lung cancer in the UK since 1950. *British Medical Journal*, 321, 323–329.

32 *Ibid.*

33 http://www.osteo.org/osteo.html

34 http://www.imaginis.com/osteoporosis/osteo_diagnose.asp

35 Rang, H. P., Dale, M. M. and Ritter, J. M., 1999. *Pharmacology*. Fourth edition. Churchill Livingstone.

36 Lee, John R, 1999. *Natural Progesterone*. Second revised edition. Jon Carpenter.

37 http://www.osteo.org

38 http://www.osteoporosis.ca

39 http://www.nos.org.uk

40 http://www.osteo.org

41 *Dietary Reference Intakes for Calcium, Phosphorus, Magnesium, Vitamin D, and Fluoride*. Report from the US Institute of Medicine.

42 http://www4.nationalacademies.org/onpi/news.nsf/0a254cd9b53e0bc585256777004e7 4d3/ f2b418098921fl9f85256774006c3b8d?Open Document

43 Bryant, H. U. and others, 1999. An estrogen receptor basis for raloxifene action in bone. *Journal of Steroid Biochemistry and Molecular Biology*, 69, 37–44.

44 Jilka, R. L. and others, 1998. Loss of estrogen upregulates osteoblastogenesis in the murine bone marrow. Evidence for autonomy from factors released during bone resorption. *Journal of Clinical Investigation*, 101, 1942–1950.

45 Sims N. A. and others, 1996. Estradiol treatment transiently increases trabecular bone volume in ovariectomized rats. *Bone*, 19, 455–461.

46 Westerlind, K. C. and others, 1993. Estrogen does not increase bone formation in growing rats. *Endocrinology*, 133, 2924–2934.

47 Smith G. R. and others, 1975. Inhibitory action of oestrogen on calcium-induced mitosis in rat bone marrow and thymus. *J Endocrinol*, 65, 45–53.

48 Vegeto, E. and others, 1999. Estrogen and progesterone induction of survival of monoblastoid cells undergoing TNF-alpha-induced apoptosis. *FASEB J.*, 13, 793–803.

49 Tomkinson, A. and others, 1998. The role of estrogen in the control of rat osteocyte apoptosis. *Journal of Bone and Mineral Research*, 13, 1243–1250.

50 *N E J of Med*, 3 Aug 1989. Reported in *WDDTY*, 4, 9.

51 *British Journal of Obstetrics and Gynaecology*, July 1987. Reported in *WDDTY*, 4, 9.

52 Writing Group for the Women's Health Initiative Investigators, 2002. Risks and benefits of estrogen plus progestin in healthy post-menopausal women. *JAMA*, 288 (3), 321–333.

53 http://www.osteo.org/osteo.html

54 Thorsen and others, 1997. *Surgery*, 122, 882–887.

55 Johnston, C. C., Peacock M. and Meunier, P., 1987. Osteomalacia as a risk factor for hip fracture in the USA. In: Christiansen, C., Johansen, J. S., Riis, B. J., editors. *Osteoporosis*. Copenhagen: Osteopress, 317–20.

56 Chapuy, M. C. and Meunier, P. J., 1996. Prevention of secondary hyperparathyroidism and hip fracture in elderly women with calcium and vitamin D3 supplements. *Osteoporosis International*, 6 (Suppl 3), 60–63.

57 Garnero, P., Hausherr, E., Chapuy, M. C. and others, 1996. Markers of bone resorption predict hip fracture in elderly women: the EPIDOS Prospective Study. *J Bone Miner Res*, 11 (10), 1531–1538.

58 Szulc, P., Chapuy, M. C., Meunier, P. J. and others, 1996. Serum undercarboxylated osteocalcin is a marker of the risk of hip fracture: a three year follow-up study. *Bone*, 18 (5), 487–488.

59 http://www.postgradmed.com/issues/1998/10_98/goddard.htm

60 Cox, Peter and Brusseau, Peggy, 1992. *Superliving: A Beginner's Guide to Medspeak*, Vermillion.

61 Rector-Page, Linda G., 1992. *Healthy Healing, 9th*, Carmel Valley: Healthy Healing Publications, 9.

Chapter 2: Bare Bones and Bags of Water

1   Johnson, D. R. Centre for Human Biology. Introductory Anatomy: Bones. http://www.leeds.ac.uk/chb/

2   Finkelman, R. B., Skinner, C. W., Plumlee, G. S. and Bunnell, J. E., 2001. Medical Geology. *Geotimes*, November 2001, 20–23. Skinner, H. Catherine W., 2001. In praise of phosphates, or why vertebrates chose apatite to mineralise their skeletal elements. *International Geological Reviews*, 42, 232–40.

3   Plant, Jane. 2001. *Your Life in Your Hands*. Paperback edition. Virgin Books.

4   Plant, Jane and Tidey, Gill. 2002. *The Plant Programme*. Paperback edition. Virgin Books.

5   Rang, H. P., Dale, M. M. and Ritter, J. M., 1999. *Pharmacology*. Fourth edition. Churchill Livingstone.

6   Lee, J. R., 1999. *Natural Progesterone*. Second revised edition. Jon Carpenter.

7   Rang, H. P., Dale, M. M. and Ritter, J. M., 1999. *Pharmacology*. Fourth edition. Churchill Livingstone.

8   *Ibid.*

9   Weinstein R. S. and others, 2000. Apoptosis and osteoporosis. *American Journal of Medicine*, 108 (2), 153–164.

10 Manolagas, S. C., 2000. Birth and death of bone cells: basic regulatory mechanisms and implications for the pathogenesis and treatment of osteoporosis. *Endocrinology Review*, 21 (2), 115–137.

11 Rodriguez, J. P., 1999. Abnormal osteogenesis in osteoporotic patients is reflected by altered mesenchymal stem cells dynamics. *Journal of Cellular Biochemistry*, 75 (3), 414–423.

12 Gazit, D. and others, 1998. Bone loss (osteopenia) in old male mice results from diminished activity and availability of TGF-beta. *J Cell Biochem*, 70 (4), 478–488.

13 Ikeda, T. and others, 1995. Age-related reduction in bone matrix protein mRNA expression in rat bone tissues: application of histomorphometry to in situ hybridization. *Bone*, 16 (1), 17–23.

14 Parfitt, A. M. and others, 1995. Relations between histologic indices of bone formation: implications for the pathogenesis of spinal osteoporosis. *Journal of Bone and Mineral Research*, 10 (3), 466–473.

15 Neidlinger-Wilke, C. and others, 1995. Human osteoblasts from younger normal and osteoporotic donors show differences in proliferation and TGF beta-release in response to cyclic strain. *Journal of Biomechanics*, 28 (12), 1411–1418.

16 Marie, P. J., 1991. Decreased DNA synthesis by cultured osteoblastic cells in eugonadal osteoporotic men with defective bone formation. *Journal of Clinical Investigation*, 88 (4), 1167–1172.

17 Byers, R. J. and others, 1997. Differential patterns of osteoblast dysfunction in trabecular bone in patients with established osteoporosis. *Journal of Clinical Pathology*, 50 (9), 760–764.

18 Mullender, M. G. and others, 1996. Osteocyte density changes in aging and osteoporosis. *Bone*, 18 (2), 109–113.

19 Ikeda, T. and others, 1995. Age-related reduction in bone matrix protein mRNA expression in rat bone tissues: application of histomorphometry to in situ hybridization. *Bone*, 16 (1), 17–23.

20 Hills, E. and others, 1989. Bone histology in young adult osteoporosis. *J Clin Pathol*, 42 (4), 391–397.

21 Kassem, M. and others, 1997. Demonstration of cellular aging and senescence in serially passaged long-term cultures of human trabecular osteoblasts. *Osteoporosis International*, 7 (6), 514–524.

22 de Vernejoul, M. C. and others, 1989. Bone remodelling in osteoporosis. *Clinical Rheumatology*, 8, Suppl. 2, 13–15.

23 Delany, A. M. and others, 2000. Osteopenia and decreased bone formation in osteonectin-deficient mice. *J Clin Invest*, 105 (7), 915–923.

24 Gazit, D. and others, 1998. Bone loss (osteopenia) in old male mice results from diminished activity and availability of TGF-beta. *J Cell Biochem*, 70 (4), 478–488.

25 Arlot, M. and others, 1984. Impaired osteoblast function in osteoporsis: comparison between calcium balance and dynamic histomorphometry. *British Medical Journal (Clinical Research Edition)*, 289 (6444), 517–520.

26 Namkung-Matthai, H. and others, 2001. Osteoporosis influences the early period of fracture healing in a rat osteoporotic model. *Bone*, 28 (1), 80–86.

27 Dunstan, C. R. and others, 1990. Bone death in hip fracture in the elderly. *Calcified Tissue International*, 47 (5), 270–275.

28 Guyton, A. C. and Hall, J. E., 2000. *Textbook of Medical Physiology*. Tenth edition. W. B. Saunders Company.

29 Rose, Steven, with Mileusnic, Radmila. 1999. *The Chemistry of Life*. Fourth (revised) edition. Penguin.

30 Modified from Table 1 in: Rose, Steven, with Mileusnic, Radmila. 1999. *The Chemistry of Life*. Fourth (revised) edition. Penguin.

31 http://www.herbsforlife.org/bufferPH.htm

32 Guyton, A. C. and Hall, J. E., 2001. *Textbook of Medical Physiology*. Tenth edition. W. B. Saunders Company.

33 Bedani, A. and DuBose, T. D., 1995. Cellular and whole-body acid-base regulation. In: *Fluid, Electrolyte and Acid Base Disorders*. Arieff, A. I. and DeFronzo, R. A., editors. Churchill Livingstone, 69–103.

34 Guyton, A. C., 1980. *Textbook of Medical Physiology*. Second edition. W. B. Saunders Co., pp. 457, 803, 853.

35 http://www.bloodph.com/research/vegetar.html

36 Rose, Steven, with Mileusnic, Radmila. 1999. *The Chemistry of Life.* Fourth (revised) edition. Penguin.

37 Bedani, A. and DuBose, T. D., 1995. Cellular and whole-body acid-base regulation. In: *Fluid, Electrolyte and Acid Base Disorders.* Arieff, A. I. and DeFronzo, R. A., editors. Churchill Livingstone, 69–103.

38 Narins, R. C., Kupi, W., Faber, M. D., Goodkin, D. A. and Dunfee, T. D., 1995. Pathophysiology, class and therapy of acid-base disorders. In: *Fluid, Electrolyte and Acid Base Disorders.* Arieff, A. I. and DeFronzo, R. A., editors. Churchill Livingstone, 104–198.

39 Berkow R., editor, 1982. *Merck Manual.* Fourteenth edition. Merck, Sharp & Dohme Research Labs, Rahwy, NJ, 945–952.

40 Guyton, A. C. and Hall, J. E., 2000. *Textbook of Medical Physiology.* Tenth edition. W. B. Saunders Company.

41 Based on http://www.chemtutor.com

42 http://wiz2.pharm.wayne.edu/module/pha413.html

43 Guyton, A. C. and Hall, J. E., 2000. *Textbook of Medical Physiology.* Tenth edition. W. B. Saunders Company.

44 Based on http://www.chemtutor.com

45 Guyton, A. C. and Hall, J. E., 2000. *Textbook of Medical Physiology.* Tenth edition. W. B. Saunders Company.

Chapter 3: Boning Up

1 Gaby, Alan R, 1994. *Preventing and reversing osteoporosis.* Rocklin, CA: Prima Publishing.

2 Plant, Jane, 2001. *Your Life in Your Hands.* Paperback edition. Virgin Books.

3 Frassetto, L. A., Todd, K. M., Morris, R. C., Jr and Sebastian, A., 2000. Worldwide incidence of hip fracture in elderly women: relation to consumption of animal and vegetable foods. *Journal of Gerontology: Medical Sciences,* 55A, 10, M585–M592.

4 Melton, L. J. III, 1995. How many women have osteoporosis now? *Journal of Bone Mineral Research,* 10, 175–177.

5 Memon, A. and others, 1998. Incidence of hip fracture in Kuwait. *International Journal of Epidemiology,* 5, 860–865.

6 Walker, A., 1965. Osteoporosis and calcium deficiency. *American Journal of Clinical Nutrition,* 16, 327.

7 Smith, R., 1966. Epidemiologic studies of osteoporosis in women of Puerto Rico and South-eastern Michigan. *Clinical Orthopaedics,* 45, 32.

8 Abelow, B. J. and others, 1992. Cross-cultural association between dietary animal protein and hip fracture: a hypothesis. *Calcified Tissue International,* 50 (1), 14–18.

9 Plant, Jane, 2001. *Your Life in Your Hands.* Paperback edition. Virgin Books.

10 *Food Balance Sheets,* 1991. Statistics Division of the Economic and Social Policy Department. Food and Agriculture Organisation of the United Nations.

11 Frassetto, L. A., Todd, K. M., Morris, R. C., Jr and Sebastian, A., 2000. Worldwide incidence of hip fracture in elderly women: relation to consumption of animal and vegetable foods. *J Geront: Med Sci,* 55A, 10, M585–M592.

12 Robbins, John, 1987. *A Diet for a New America.* Stillpoint.

13 http://www.milksucks.com/osteo.html

14 *American Journal of Epidemiology,* 1994.

15 FAO database on the internet; http://www.fao.org/Statistical Database/Food Balance Sheet Reports. Hong Kong has been removed from the database since the unification with China.

16 Paspati, I. and others, 1998. Hip fracture epidemiology in Greece during 1977–1992. *Calcif Tissue Int,* 62 (6), 542–547.

17 FAO database on the internet: http://www.fao.org/Statistical Database/Food Balance
    Sheet Reports. Hong Kong has been removed from the database since the unification
    with China.

18 Lau, E. M. and Cooper, C., 1993. Epidemiology and prevention of osteoporosis in
    urbanized Asian populations. *Osteoporosis*, 3, suppl. 1, 23–26.

19 Ho, S. C. and others, 1999. The prevalence of osteoporosis in the Hong Kong Chinese
    female population. *Maturitas*, 1999 Aug 16, 32 (3), 171–178.

20 Versluis, R. G. and others, 1999. Prevalence of osteoporosis in post-menopausal women
    in family practise (in Dutch). *Nederlands Tijdschrift voor Geneeskunde*, 143 (1), 20–24.

21 Oden, A. and others, 1998. Lifetime risk of hip fractures is underestimated.
    Osteoporosis International, 8 (6), 599–603.

22 Smeets-Goevaars, C. G. and others, 1998. The prevalence of low bone-mineral density
    in Dutch perimenopausal women: the Eindhoven perimenopausal osteoporosis study.
    Osteoporosis Int, 8 (5), 404–409.

23 Lippuner, K. O. and others, 1997. Incidence and direct medical costs of hospitalizations
    due to osteoporotic fractures in Switzerland. *Osteoporosis Int*, 7 (5), 414–425.

24 Lips, P., 1997. Epidemiology and predictors of fractures associated with osteoporosis.
    American Journal of Medicine, 103 (2A), 3S–8S; discussion 8S–11S.

25 Parkkari, J. and others, 1996. Secular trends in osteoporotic pelvic fractures in Finland:
    number and incidence of fractures in 1970–1991 and prediction for the future. *Calcif
    Tissue Int*, 59 (2), 79–83.

26 Nydegger, V. and others, 1991. Epidemiology of fractures of the proximal femur in
    Geneva; incidence, clinical and social aspects. *Osteoporosis Int*, 2 (1), 42–47.

27 Van Hemert, A. M. and others, 1990. Prediction of osteoporotic fractures in the general
    population by a fracture risk score. A 9-year follow up among middle aged women. *Am
    J Epidemiol*, 132 (1), 123–135.

28 Lau, E. M. and others, 1993. Admission rates for hip fracture in Australia in the last
    decade. The New South Wales scene in a world perspective. *Medical Journal of
    Australia*, 158 (9), 604–606.

29 Fujita, T. and Fukase, M., 1992. Comparison of osteoporosis and calcium intake
    between Japan and the United States. *Proceedings of the Society for Experimental Biology
    and Medicine*, 200 (2), 149–152.

30 Bauer, R. L., 1988. Ethnic differences in hip fracture: a reduced incidence in Mexican
    Americans. *Am J Epidemiol*, 1988 Jan, 127 (1), 145–149.

31 Kessenich C. R., 2000. Osteoporosis and African-American women. *Women's Health
    Issues*, 10 (6), 300–304.

32 Bwanahali, K. and others, 1992. Etiological aspects of low back pain in rheumatic
    patients in Kinshasa (Zaire). Apropos of 169 cases (in French). *Revue du Rhumatisme et
    des Maladies Osteo-articulaires*, 59 (4), 253–257.

33 Barss, P., 1985. Fractured hips in rural Melanesians: a nonepidemic. *Tropical and
    Geographical Medicine*, 37 (2), 156–159.

34 Mijiyawa, M. A. and others, 1991. Rheumatic diseases in hospital outpatients in Lome
    (in French). *Rev Rhum Mal Osteoartic*, 58 (5), 349–354.

35 Davis, J. W. and others, 1999. Ethnic, anthropometric, and lifestyle associations with
    regional variations in peak bone mass. *Calcif Tissue Int*, 1999 Aug, 65 (2), 100–105.

36 Ulrich, C. M. and others, 1999. Lifetime physical activity is associated with bone
    mineral density in premenopausal women. *Journal of Women's Health*, 1999 Apr, 8 (3),
    365–375.

37 Boot, A. M. and others, 1997. Bone mineral density in children and adolescents:
    relation to puberty, calcium intake, and physical activity. *Journal of Clinical
    Endocrinology Metabolism*, 1997 Jan, 82 (1), 57–62.

38 Hu, J. F. and others, 1993. Dietary calcium and bone density among middle-aged and elderly women in China. *Am J Clin Nutr*, 1993 Aug, 58 (2), 219–227.

39 Dargent-Molina, P. and 7 others, for the EPIDOS Group, 1996. Fall-related factors and the risk of hip fracture: the EPIDOS prospective study. *The Lancet*, 348, 145–149.

40 Cummings, S. R. and others, for the Study of Osteoporotic Fractures Research Group, 1995. Risk factors for hip fracture in white women. *New England Journal of Medicine*, 332, 767–773.

41 Sellmeyer, D. E., Stone, K. S., Sebastian, A. and Cummings, S. R. 2001. A high ratio of dietary animal to vegetable protein increases the rate of bone loss and the risk of fracture in post-menopausal women. *Am J Clin Nutr*, 73, 118–122.

42 *American Journal of Clinical Nutrition*, 2000.

43 Rang, H. P., Dale, M. M. and Ritter, J. M., 1999. *Pharmacology*. Fourth edition. Churchill Livingstone.

44 Schwartz, A. V. and others, 1999. International variation in the incidence of hip fractures: cross-national project on osteoporosis for the World Health Organization Program for Research on Ageing. *Osteoporosis Int*, 9 (3), 242–253.

45 Rowe, S. M. and others, 1993. An epidemiological study of hip fracture in Honan, Korea. *International Orthopaedics*, 17 (3), 139–143.

46 Pritikin, N., quoted in *Vegetarian Times*, issue 43, 22.

47 Walker, A., 1965. Osteoporosis and calcium deficiency. *Am J Clin Nut*, 16, 327.

48 Smith, R., 1966. Epidemiological studies of osteoporosis in women of Puerto Rico and south-eastern Michigan. *Clinical Orthpaedics*, 45, 32.

49 Mazees, R., 1974. Bone mineral content of North Alaskan Eskimos. *American Journal of Clinical Nutrition*, 27, 916.

50 http://www.4.waisays.com

51 Erben, R. G. and others, 2000. Androgen deficiency induces high turnover osteopenia in aged male rats: a sequential histomorphometric study. *J Bone Miner Res*, 15, 1085–1098.

52 Yeh, K. and others, 1996. Ovariectomy-induced high turnover in cortical bone is dependent on pituary hormone in rats. *Bone*, 18, 443–540.

53 Garnero, P. and others, 1996. Increased bone turnover in late post-menopausal women is a major determinant of osteoporosis. *J Bone Miner Res*, 11, 337–349.

54 Taguchi, Y. and others, 1998. Interleukin-6-type cytokines stimulate mesenchymal progenitor differentiation toward the osteoblastic lineage. *Proceedings of the Association of American Physicians*, 110 (6), 559–574.

55 Jilka, R. L. and others, 1998. Loss of estrogen upregulates osteoblastogenesis in the murine bone marrow. Evidence for autonomy from factors released during bone resorption. *Journal of Clinical Investigation*, 101 (9), 1942–1950.

56 Tau, K. R. and others, 1998. Estrogen regulation of a transforming growth factor-beta inducible early gene that inhibits deoxyribonucleic acid synthesis in human osteoblasts. *Endocrinology*, 139 (3), 1346–1353.

57 Hietala, E. L., 1993. The effect of ovariectomy on periosteal bone formation and bone resorption in adult rats. *Journal of Bone and Mineral Research*, 20 (1), 57–65.

58 Egrise, D. and others, 1992. Bone blood flow and in vitro proliferation of bone marrow and trabecular bone osteoblast-like cells in ovariectomized rats. *Calcif Tissue Int*, 50 (4), 336–341.

59 Jilka, R. L. and others, 1998. Osteoblast programmed cell death (apoptosis): modulation by growth factors and cytokines. *J Bone Miner Res*, 13 (5), 793–802.

60 Mogi, M. and others, 1999. Involvement of nitric oxide and biopterin in proinflammatory cytokine-induced apoptotic cell death in mouse osteoblastic cell line MC3T3-E1. *Biochemical Pharmacology*, 58 (4), 649–654.

61 Kobayashi, E. T. and others, 1999. Force-induced rapid changes in cell fate at midpalatal suture cartilage of growing rats. *Journal of Dental Research*, 78 (9), 1495–1504.

62 O'Brien, K. O. and others, 1996. Increased efficiency of calcium absorption from the rectum and distal colon of humans. *Am J Clin Nutr*, 63 (4), 579–583.

63 http://www.4.waisays.com/

64 Peterson C. A. and others, 1995. Alterations in calcium intake on peak bone mass in the female rat. *J Bone Miner Res*, 10 (1), 81–95.

65 http://www.4.waisays.com

66 Pazzaglia, U. E., 1990. Experimental osteoporosis in the rat induced by a hypocalcic diet. *Italian Journal of Orthopaedics and Traumatology*, 16 (2), 257–265.

67 http://www.internethealthlibrary.com/Health-problems/Osteoporosis-researchDiet&Lifestyle.htm#Animal%20Protein

68 http://www.4.waisays.com

69 Mazzuoli, G. F. and others, 1993. Hip fracture in Italy: Epidemiology and preventive efficacy of bone active drugs. *Bone*, 14, suppl., 581–584.

70 Lips, P., 1997. Epidemiology and predictors of fractures associated with osteoporosis. *Am J Med*, 103 (2A), 3S–8S; discussion 8S–11S.

71 FAO database on the internet: www.fao.org/Statistical Database/Food Balance Sheet Reports. Hong Kong has been removed from the database since the unification with China.

72 *Ibid.*

73 Memon, A. and others, 1998. Incidence of hip fracture in kuwait. *Int J Epidemiol*, 5, 860–865.

74 Ghannam, N. N. and others, 1999. Bone mineral density of the spine and femur in healthy Saudi females: relation to vitamin D status, pregnancy, and lactation. *Calcif Tissue Int*, 1999 Jul, 65 (1), 23–28.

75 http://www.4.waisays.com

76 Sairanen S. and others, 2000. Bone mass and markers of bone and calcium metabolism in post-menopausal women treated with 1,25-dihydroxyvitamin D (Calcitriol) for four years. *Calcif Tissue Int*, 67 (2), 122–127.

77 Gurlek, A. and others, 1997. Comparison of calcitriol treatment with etidronate-calcitriol and calcitonin-calcitriol combinations in Turkish women with post-menopausal osteoporosis: a prospective study. *Calcif Tissue Int*, 61 (1), 39–43.

78 Giunta, D. L., 1998. Dental changes in hypervitaminosis D. *Oral Surgery, Oral Medicine, Oral Pathology, Oral Radiology and Endodontics*, 85 (4), 410–413.

79 Uehlinger, P. and others, 1998. Differential diagnosis of hypercalcemia – a retrospective study of 46 dogs. (duitst.) *Schweizer Archiv für Tierheilkunde*, 140 (5), 188–197.

80 Qin, X. and others, 1997. Altered phosphorylation of a 91-kDa protein in particulate fractions of rat kidney after protracted 1,25-dihydroxyvitamin D3 or estrogen treatment. *Archives of Biochemistry and Biophysics*, 348 (2), 239–246.

81 Niederhoffer, N. and others, 1997. Calcification of medical elastic fibers and aortic elasticity. *Hypertension*, 29 (4), 999–1006.

82 Selby, P. L. and others, 1995. Vitamin D intoxication causes hypercalcemia by increased bone resorption with responds to pamidronate. *Clin Endocrinol* (Oxford), 43 (5), 531–536.

83 Ito, M. and others, 1987. Dietary magnesium effect on swine coronary atherosclerosis induced by hypervitaminosis D. *Acta Pathologica Japonica*, 37 (6), 955–964.

84 Frassetto, L. A., Todd, K. M., Morris, R. C., Jr and Sebastian, A., 2000. Worldwide incidence of hip fracture in elderly women: relation to consumption of animal and vegetable foods. *J Geront: Med Sci*, 55A, 10, M585–M592.

85 Abelow, B. J., Holford, T. R., and Insogna, K. L., 1992. Cross-cultural association between dietary and animal protein and hip fracture: a hypothesis. *Calcif Tissue Int*, 50, 14–18.

86 Frassetto, L. A., Todd, K. M., Morris, R. C., Jr and Sebastian, A., 2000. Worldwide incidence of hip fracture in elderly women: relation to consumption of animal and vegetable foods. *J Geront: Med Sci*, 55A, 10, M585–M592.

87 *Ibid*.

88 Chalmers, J., 1970. Geographic variations of senile osteoporosis. *Journal of Bone & Joint Surgery*, 52B, 667.

89 Walker, A., 1972. Calcium retention in the adult human male as affected by protein intake. *Journal of Nutrition*, 102, 1297.

90 http://www.milksucks.com/osteo.html

91 Heaney, R. P., 1993. *Journal of the American Dietetic Association*.

92 Sellmeyer, D. E., Stone, K. S., Sebastian, A. and Cummings, S. R. 2001. A high ratio of dietary animal to vegetable protein increases the rate of bone loss and the risk of fracture in post-menopausal women. *Am J Clin Nutr*, 73, 118–122.

93 Hawkins, H. F., 1947. *Applied Nutrition*. International College of Applied Nutrition. La Habra, California.

94 Beisel, W. R., 1990. Nutrition and infection. In: *Nutritional Biochemistry and Metabolism*. Linder, M., editor. Elsevier. New York, 507–542.

95 Bedani, A., DuBose, T. D., 1995. Cellular and whole-body acid-base regulation. In: *Fluid, Electrolyte and Acid Base Disorders*. Arieff, A. I. and DeFronzo, R. A., editors. Churchill Livingstone. New York, 69–103.

96 Hawkins, H. F., 1947. *Applied Nutrition*. International College of Applied Nutrition. La Habra, California.

97 Fox, Douglas, 2001. Hard cheese. *New Scientist*, 15 December 2001, 42–45.

98 http://www.milksucks.com/osteo.html

Chapter 4: Balancing for Your Bones

1 Fox, Douglas, 2001. Hard cheese. *New Scientist*, 15 December 2001, 42–45.

2 *Ibid*.

3 *Ibid*.

4 http://www.internethealthlibrary.com

5 Marsh, A. G., Sanchez, T. V., Michelsen, O., Chaffee, F. L. and Fagal, S. M., 1988. *American Journal of Clinical Nutrition*, 48 (3 Suppl), 837–841.

6 http://www.internethealthlibrary.com

7 http://pacificcoast.net/ ~ rustym/articles/PH.html

8 Remer, T. and Manz, F., 1995. Potential renal acid load of foods and its influence on urine pH. *Journal of the American Dietetic Association*, 95, No. 7, 791–797.

9 Fox, Douglas, 2001. Hard Cheese. *New Scientist*, 15 December 2001, 42–45

10 http://pacificcoast.net/~ rustym/articles/PH.html

11 Willis, Amrit, 2001. *Solving the Interstitial Cystitis Puzzle*. Holistic Life Enterprises. Excerpted at http://holisticnurse.com/books/ic/ic-preface.shtml

12 Lark, Susan and Richards, James A., 2000. *The Chemistry of Success*. San Francisco: Bay Books, 55.

13 *Ibid*.

14 http://pacificcoast.net/~ rustym/articles/PH.html

15 Baroody, Theodore A. Jr, 1993. *Alkalize or Die*. Waynesville, NC: Eclectic Press, 21–22.

16 Frassetto, L. A., Todd, K. M., Morris, R. C., Jr and Sebastian, A., 2000. Worldwide incidence of hip fracture in elderly women: relation to consumption of animal and vegetable foods. *Journal of Gerontology: Medical Sciences*, 55A, 10, M585–M592.

17 Sellmeyer, D. E., Stone, K. S., Sebastian, A. and Cummings, S. R. 2001. A high ratio of dietary animal to vegetable protein increases the rate of bone loss and the risk of fracture in post-menopausal women. *Am J Clin Nutr*, 73, 118–122.

18 Blatherwick, N. R., 1914. The specific role of foods in relation to the composition of the urine. *Archives of Internal Medicine*, 14, 409–450.

19 Hu, J-F., Zhao, X-H., Parpia, B. and Campbell, T. C., 1993. Dietary intakes and urinary excretion of calcium and acids: a cross-sectional study of women in China. *Am J Clin Nutr* 58, 398–406.

20 Kurtz, I., Maher, T., Hulter, H. N., Schambelan, M. and Sebastian, A., 1983. Effect of diet on plasma acid-base composition in normal humans. *Kidney International*, 24, 670–680.

21 Frassetto, L., Morris, R. C., Jr and Sebastian, A., 1996. Effect of age on blood acid-base composition in adult humans: role of age-related renal functional decline. *American Journal of Physiology*, 271, 1114–1122.

22 Kurtz, I., Maher, T., Hulter, H. N., Schambelan, M. and Sebastian, A., 1983. Effect of diet on plasma acid-base composition in normal humans. *Kidney Int*, 24, 670–680.

23 *Ibid*.

24 Lennon, E. J., Lemann, J., Jr and Litzow, J. R., 1966. The effect of diet and stool composition on the net external acid balance of normal subjects. *Journal of Clinical Investigation*, 45, 1601–1607.

25 Kurtz, I., Maher, T., Hulter, H. N., Schambelan, M. and Sebastian, A., 1983. Effect of diet on plasma acid-base composition in normal humans. *Kidney Int*, 24, 670–680.

26 Lennon, E. J., Lemann, J., Jr and Litzow, J. R., 1966. The effect of diet and stool composition on the net external acid balance of normal subjects. *J Clin Invest*, 45, 1601–1607.

27 Lemann, J. Jr, Litzow, J. R. and Lennon, E. J., 1966. The effect of chronic acid loads in normal man: further evidence for participation of bone mineral in the defense against chronic metabolic acidosis. *J Clin Invest*, 45, 1608–1614.

28 Lemann, J., Jr, Lennon, E. J., Goodman, A. D., Litzow, J. R. and Relman, A. S., 1965. The net balance of acid in subjects given large loads of acid or alklali. *J Clin Invest*, 44, 507–517.

29 Green, J. and Kleeman, C. R., 1991. The role of bone in regulation of systemic acid-base balance. *Kidney Int*, 39, 9–26.

30 Wachman, A. and Bernstein, D. S., 1968. Diet and osteoporosis. *Lancet*, 1, 958–959.

31 Barzel, U. S. and Massey, L. K., 1998. Excess dietary protein can adversely affect bone. *Journal of Nutrition*, 128, 1051–1053.

32 Sebastian, A., Harris, S. T., Ottaway, J. H., Todd, K. M. and Morris, R. C. Jr, 1994. Improved mineral balance and skeletal metabolism in postmenopausal women treated with potassium bicarbonate. *New England Journal of Medicine*, 330, 1776–1781.

33 Rector, F. C., 1973. Acidification of the urine. *Handbook of Physiology Section 8: Renal Physiology*. Orloff, J., Berliner, R. W. and Fieger, S., editors. American Physiological Society. Washington DC, 431–454.

34 Ensminger, A. H., Ensminger, M. E., Konlande, J. E. and Robsin, J. R. K., 1994, *Foods and Nutrition Encyclopedia*. Second edition. Boca Raton, Florida: CRC Press, 6–7, 41.

35 Read, A. and Ilstrup, C., 1967. *A Diet/Recipe Guide Based on the Edgar Cayce Readings*. Virginia Beach, Va: ARE Press.

36 Ensminger, A. H., Ensminger, M. E., Konlande, J. E. and Robsin, J. R. K., 1994. *Foods and Nutrition Encyclopedia*. Second edition. Boca Raton, Florida: CRC Press, 6–7, 41.

37 Read, A. and Ilstrup, C., 1967. *A Diet/Recipe Guide Based on the Edgar Cayce Readings*. Virginia Beach, Va: ARE Press.

38 Rector, F. C., 1973. Acidification of the urine. *Handbook of Physiology Section 8: Renal*

Physiology. Orloff, J., Berliner, R. W. and Fieger, S., editors. American Physiological Society. Washington DC, 431–454.

39 Ensminger, A. H., Ensminger, M. E., Konlande, J. E. and Robsin, J. R. K., 1994. *Foods and Nutrition Encyclopedia*. Second edition. Boca Raton, Florida: CRC Press, 6–7, 41.

40 Hawkins, H. F., 1947. *Applied Nutrition*. La Habra, California: International College of Applied Nutrition.

41 Remer, T. and Manz, F. 1995. Potential renal acid load of foods and its influence on urine pH. *J Am Diet Assoc*, 95, No. 7, 791–797.

42 Dwyer, J., Foulkes, E., Evans, M. and Ausman, L., 1985. Acid/alkaline ash diets: time for assessment and change. *J Am Diet Assoc*, 85, 841–845.

43 Remer, T. and Manz, F. 1994. Estimation of the renal net acid excretion by adults consuming diets containing variable amounts of protein. *Am J Clin Nutr*, 59, 1356–1361.

44 Dwyer, J., Foulkes, E., Evans, M. and Ausman, L., 1985. Acid/alkaline ash diets: time for assessment and change. *J Am Diet Assoc*, 85, 841–845.

45 Remer, T. and Manz, F. 1994. Estimation of the renal net acid excretion by adults consuming diets containing variable amounts of protein. *Am J Clin Nutr*, 59, 1356–1361.

46 Siener, R. and Hesse, A., 1993. Einfluß verschiedener Kostformen auf die Harnzusammensetzung und das Kalziumoxalat-Steinbildungsrisiko. *Z Ernahrungswiss*, 32, 46–55.

47 Remer, T. and Manz, F., 1995. Dietary protein as a modulator of the renal net acid excretion capacity: evidence that an increased protein intake improves the capability of the kidney to excrete ammonium. *Journal of Nutritional Biochemistry*, 6 (8), 431–437.

48 *Ibid.*

49 Remer, T. and Manz, F., 1995. Potential renal acid load of foods and its influence on urine pH. *J Am Diet Assoc*, 95, 791–797, Table 3.

50 Sellmeyer, D. E., Stone, K. S., Sebastian, A. and Cummings, S. R. 2001. A high ratio of dietary animal to vegetable protein increases the rate of bone loss and the risk of fracture in post-menopausal women. *Am J Clin Nutr*, 73, 118–122.

51 Langendorf, H., 1963. Säure-Basen-Gleichgewicht und chronische acidogene und alkalogene Ernährung. *Z Ernahrungswiss*, 2 (suppl), 1–33.

52 Fox, Douglas, 2001. Hard Cheese. *New Scientist*, 15 December 2001, 42–45.

53 Langendorf, H., 1963. Säure-Basen-Gleichgewicht und chronische acidogene und alkalogene Ernährung. *Z Ernahrungswiss*, 2 (suppl), 1–33.

54 Gonick, H. C., Goldberg, G. and Mulcare, D., 1968. Reexamination of the acid-ash content of several diets. *Am J Clin Nutr*, 21, 898–903.

55 Dwyer, J., Foulkes, E., Evans, M. and Ausman, L., 1985. Acid/alkaline ash diets: time for assessment and change. *J Am Diet Assoc*, 85, 841–845.

56 Remer, T. and Manz, F., 1995. Dietary protein as a modulator of the renal net acid excretion capacity: evidence that an increased protein intake improves the capability of the kidney to excrete ammonium. *J Nutr Biochem*, 6 (8), 431–437.

57 Remer, T. and Manz, F., 1994. Estimation of the renal net acid excretion by adults consuming diets containing variable amounts of protein. *Am J Clin Nutr*, 59, 1356–1361.

58 Manz, F., Vacsei, P. and Wesch, H. 1984. Renale Säureausscheidung und renale Molenlast bei gesunden Kindern und Erwachsenen. *Monatsschr Kinderheilkd*, 132, 163–167.

59 Sebastian, A., Harris, S. T., Ottaway, J. H., Todd, K. M. and Morris, R. C. Jr, 1994. Improved mineral balance and skeletal metabolism in postmenopauisal women treated with potassium bicarbonate. *N E J of Med*, 330, 1776–1781.

60 Remer, T. and Manz, F., 1994. Estimation of the renal net acid excretion by adults consuming diets containing variable amounts of protein. *Am J Clin Nutr*, 59, 1356–1361.

61 Remer, T. and Manz, F., 1995. Dietary protein as a modulator of the renal net acid excretion capacity: evidence that an increased protein intake improves the capability of the kidney to excrete ammonium. *J Nutr Biochem*, 6 (8), 431–437.

62 Siener, R. and Hesse, A., 1993. Einfluβ verschiedener Kostformen auf die Harnzusammensetzung und das Kalziumoxalat-Steinbildungsrisiko. *Z Ernahrungswiss*, 32, 46–55.

63 Manz, F. and Schmidt, H., 1992. Retrospective approach to explain growth retardation and urolithiasis in a child with long-term nutritional acid loading. (in German) *Z Ernahrungswiss*, 31, 121–129.

64 Lemann, J., 1993. Composition of the diet and calcium kidney stones. *N E J of Med*, 328, 880–881.

65 Hasling, C., Sondergaard, K., Charles, P. and Mosekilde, L., 1992. Calcium metabolism in post-menopausal women is determined by dietary calcium and coffee intake. *J Nutr*, 122, 1119–1122.

66 Hawkins, H. F., 1947. *Applied Nutrition*. La Habra, California: International College of Applied Nutrition.

67 Pennington, J. A. T. and Wilson, D. B., 1990. Daily intakes of nine nutritional elements: analyzed vs calculated values. *J Am Diet Assoc*, 90, 375–381.

68 World Health Organisation, 1996. *Trace Elements in Human Nutrition and Health*. World Health Organisation.

69 e.g. *New England Journal of Medicine*, 1998, 339, 1112–1120.

70 http://www.nutrimed.com/OSTEO.HTM

71 Campbell, T. C. and Junshi, C., 1994. Diet and chronic degenerative disease perspectives from China. *A J Clin Nutr*, 59, suppl, 1153S–1161S.

72 http://members.tripod.com/-charles_W/copper.html

73 World Health Organisation, 1996. *Trace Elements in Human Nutrition and Health*. World Health Organisation.

74 Grand Forks Human Nutrition Research Center. http://www.gfhnrc.ars.usda.gov/News/nws0001a.htm

75 Milne, D. B., Klevay, L. M. and Hunt, J. R., 1988. Effects of ascorbic acid supplements and a diet marginal in copper on indices of copper nutriture in women. *Nutrition Research*, 8, 865–873.

76 Jacob, R. A. and others, 1987. Effect of varying ascorbic acid intakes on copper absorption and ceruloplasmin levels in young men. *J Nutr*, 117, 2109–2115.

77 Underwood, E. J., 1977. *Trace Elements in Human and Animal Nutrition*. Fourth edition. Academic Press. 56–108.

78 Snedeker, S. M., Smith, S. A. and Greger, J. L. 1982. Effect of dietary calcium and phosphorus levels on the utilisation of iron, copper and zinc by adult males. *J Nutr*, 112, 136–143.

79 Strain, J. J., 1988. *Med-Hypotheses*, 27 (4), 333–338.

80 http://www.nutrimed.com/OSTEO.HTM

81 Fincham, J. E., van Rensberg, S. J. and Marasas, W. F. O., 1981. Mseleni joint disease – a manganese deficiency? *South African Medical Journal*, 60, 445–447.

82 Soman, S. D., 1969. Daily intake of some major and trace elements. *Health Physics*, 17, 35–40.

83 http://www.nutrimed.com/OSTEO.HTM

84 *Ibid.*

85 Lee, John R., 1999. *Natural Progesterone*. Second revised edition. Jon Carpenter.

86 http://www.nutrimed.com/OSTEO.HTM

Chapter 5: The 'Osteoporosis Plant Programme' – The Food Factors

1 Plant, Jane, 2001. *Your Life in Your Hands*. Paperback edition. Virgin Books.
2 Plant, Jane and Tidey, Gill, 2002. *The Plant Programme*. Paperback edition. Virgin Books.
3 Brundtland, G. H., 1987. *World Commission on Environment and Development: Our Common Future*. Oxford: Oxford University Press.
4 Fox, Douglas, 2001. Hard Cheese. *New Scientist*, 15 December 2001, 42–45.
5 From papers by T. Colin Campbell and Chen Junshi on diet and chronic degenerative disease, published in 1994.
6 Jacobs, M. N. and others, 2002. *Environmental Science and Technology*, 36, 2797–2805.
7 Heaney, R. P. and Recker, R. R., 1982. Effects of nitrogen, phosphorus, and caffeine on calcium balance in women. *Journal of Laboratory and Clinical Medicine*, 99, 1, 46–55.

Chapter 6: Lifestyle Factors

1 Milne, D. B., Klevay, L. M. and Hunt, J. R., 1988. Effects of ascorbic acid supplements and a diet marginal in copper on indices of copper nutriture in women. *Nutrition Research*, 8, 865–873.
2 Jacob, R. A. and others, 1987. Effect of varying ascorbic acid intakes on copper absorption and ceruloplasmin levels in young men. *Journal of Nutrition*, 117, 2109–2115.
3 Underwood, E. J., 1977. *Trace Elements in Human and Animal Nutrition*. Fourth edition. Academic Press, 56–108.
4 Snedeker, S. M., Smith, S. A. and Greger, J. L., 1982. Effect of dietary calcium and phosphorus levels on the utilisation of iron, copper and zinc by adult males. *J Nutr*, 112, 136–143.
5 World Health Organisation, 1996. *Trace Elements in Human Nutrition and Health*. World Health Organisation.
6 http://www.cc.nih.gov/ccc/supplements/vitdref.html
7 Institute of Medicine, Food and Nutrition Board, 1999. *Dietary Reference Intakes: Calcium, Phosphorus, Magnesium, Vitamin D and Fluoride*. National Academy Press, Washington, DC.
8 Chapuy, M. C., Arlot, M. E., Duboeuf, F., Brun, J., Crouzet, B., Arnaud, S., Delmas, P. D. and Meunier, P. J., 1992. Vitamin D3 and calcium to prevent hip fractures in elderly women. *New England Journal of Medicine*, 327, 1637–1642.
9 MacLaughlin, J., and Holick, M. F., 1985. Aging decreases the capacity of human skin to produce vitamin D3. *Journal of Clinical Investigation*, 76, 1536–1538.
10 Holick, M. F., Matsuoka, L. Y., and Wortsman, J., 1989. Age, vitamin D, and solar ultraviolet. *Lancet*, 2, 1104–1105.
11 Need, A. G., Morris, H. A., Horowitz, M., and Nordin, C., 1993. Effects of skin thickness, age, body fat, and sunlight on serum 25-hydroxyvitamin D. *American Journal of Clinical Nutrition*, 58, 882–885.
12 Reid, I. R., 1998. The roles of calcium and vitamin D in the prevention of osteoporosis. *Endocrinology and Metabolism Clinics of North America*, 27, 389–398.
13 Dawson-Hughes, B., Harris, S. S., Krall, E. A., Dallal, G. E., Falconer G. and Green, C. L., 1995. Rates of bone loss in post-menopausal women randomly assigned to one of two dosages of vitamin D. *Am J Clin Nutr*, 61, 1140–1145.
14 Reid, I. R., 1998. The roles of calcium and vitamin D in the prevention of osteoporosis. *Endocrinol Metab Clin North Am*, 27, 389–398.
15 Reid, I. R., 1996. Therapy of osteoporosis: Calcium, vitamin D, and exercise. *American Journal of Medical Science*, 312, 278–286.
16 Veith, R., 1999. Vitamin D supplementation, 25-hydroxyvitamin D concentrations, and safety. *J Am Clin Nutr*, 69, 842–856.

17 Chesney, R. W., 1989. Vitamin D: Can an upper limit be defined? *J Nutr*, 119 (12 Suppl), 1825–1828.

18 http://www.cc.nih.gov/ccc/supplements/vitdref.html

19 Retailers forced to act over dioxins in fish oils. *ENDS Report*, 330, July 2002, 7.

20 Chu, N. F. and others, 2001. Plasma leptin concentrations and four-year weight gain among US men. *International Journal of Obesity and Related Metabolic Disorders*, 25 (3), 346–353.

21 Szymczak, E. and others, 2001. The role of leptin in human obesity. *Medycyny Wieku Rozwojowego*, 5 (1), 17–26.

22 Hu, F. B. and others, 2001. Leptin concentrations in relation to overall fat adiposity, fat distribution, and blood pressure in a rural Chinese population. *Int J Obes Relat Disord*, 25 (1), 121–125.

23 Bahceci, M. and others, 1999. The effect of high-fat diet on the development of obesity and serum leptin level in rats. *Eating and Weight Disorders*, 4 (3), 128–132.

24 Milewicz, A. and others, 2000. Plasma insulin, cholecystokinin, galanin, neuropeptide Y and leptin levels in obese women with and without type 2 diabetes mellitus. *Int J Obes Relat Disord*, 24, Suppl 2, S152–153.

25 Nakamura, M. and others, 2000. Association between basal serum and leptin levels and changes in abdominal fat distribution during weight loss. *Journal of Atherosclerosis and Thrombosis*, 6 (1), 28–32.

26 Bunger, L. and others, 1999. Leptin levels in lines of mice developed by long-term divergent selection on fat content. *Genetical Research*, 73 (1), 37–44.

27 Burguera, B. and others, 2001. Leptin reduces ovariectomy-induced bone loss in rats. *Endocrinology*, 142 (8), 3546–3553.

28 Takeda, S. and others, 2001. Central control of bone formation. *Journal of Bone Mineral Metabolism*, 19 (3), 195–198.

29 Anselme, K. and others, 2000. Comparative study of the in vitro characteristics of osteoblasts from paralytic and non-paralytic children. *Spinal Cord*, 38 (10), 622–629.

30 Ducy, P. and others, 2000. Leptin inhibits bone formation through a hypothalamic relay: a central control of bone mass. *Cell*, 100 (2), 197–207.

31 http://www.fda.gov/fdac/features/2001/401_food.html

32 http://www.ifst.org/hottop19.htm

33 Taylor, S. L., 1992. Chemistry and detection of food allergens. *Food Technology*, 46 (5), 146–152.

34 http://www.ifst.org/hottop19.htm

35 Martin, Peter, 2002. Milk: Nectar or poison? *Sunday Times Magazine*, July 21, 2002.

36 http://news.bbc.co.uk/1/hi/health/713698.stm

37 Lee, John R., 1999. *Natural Progesterone*. Second revised edition. Jon Carpenter.

38 Writing Group for the Women's Health Initiative Investigators. 2002. Risks and benefits of estrogen plus progestin in healthy post-menopausal women. *Journal of the American Medical Association*, 288, (3), 321–333.

39 Kurzer, M. S. and Xu, X., 1999. Dietary phytoestrogens. *Annual Reviews of Nutrition*, 17, 353–381.

40 The Royal Society, 2000. Endocrine-disrupting chemicals. *Document* 06/00. The Royal Society.

41 Lee, John R., 1999. *Natural Progesterone*. Second revised edition. Jon Carpenter.

42 Phipps, W. R., Martini, M. C., Lampe, J. W., Slavin, J. L. and Kurzer, M. S., 1993. Effect of flax seed ingestion on the menstrual cycle. *Journal of Clinical Endocrinology Metabolism*, 77, 5, November 1993, 1215–1219.

43 http://www.flax.com.fda

44 Lee, John R., 1999. *Natural Progesterone*. Second revised edition. Jon Carpenter.

45 http://www.bewellstaywell.com/osteoporosis.htm

46 Ernst, E. (editor), 2001. *The Desktop Guide to Complementary and Alternative Medicine: an evidence based approach*. Mosby.

47 Rutherford, O. M. and others, 1992. The relationship of muscle and bone loss and activity levels with age in women. *Age and Ageing*, 21 (4), 286–293.

48 Ernst, E., 1998. Exercise for female osteoporosis. A systematic review of randomised clinical trials. *Sports Medicine*, 25, 359–368.

49 Wolff, I. and others, 1999. The effect of exercise training programs on bone mass: a meta-analysis of published control trials in pre- and post-menopausal women. *Osteoporosis International*, 9, 1–12.

50 Lee, J. R., 1999. *Natural Progesterone*. Second revised edition. Jon Carpenter.

51 Meyer, T. and others, 1999. Identification of apoptotic cell death in distraction osteogenesis. *Cell Biology International*, 23 (6), 439–446.

52 Landry, P. and others, 1997. Apoptosis is coordinately regulated with osteoblast formation during bone healing. *Tissue and Cell*, 29 (4), 413–419.

53 Cromer, B. and others, 2000. Adolescents: at increased risk for osteoporosis? *Clinical Pediatrics (Phila)*, 39 (10), 565–574.

54 Judex S. and others, 2000. Does the mechanical milieu associated with high-speed running lead to adaptive changes in diaphyseal growing bone?, Feb 2000 Bone, 26 (2), 153–159.

55 Kaastad, T. S. and others, 1996. Training increases the in vivo fracture strength in osteoporotic bone. Protection by muscle contraction examined in rat tibiae. *Acta Orthopaedica Scandinavica*, 67 (4), 371–376.

56 http://www.medicinenet.com/script/main/art.asp?articlekey = 6860&rd = 1

57 Katz, W. A. with Sherman, C., 1998. Exercise for osteoporosis. *The Physician and Sportsmedicine*, 26, 2. http://www.physsportsmed.com/issues/1998/02feb/katzpa.htm.

58 http://www.focusonosteoporosis.com/script/main/art.asp?articlekey = 6860&rd = 1

59 Katz, W. A. with Sherman, C., 1998. Exercise for osteoporosis. *The Physician and Sportsmedicine*, 26, 2. http://www.physsportsmed.com/issues/1998/02feb/katzpa.htm.

60 Ernst, E. (editor), 2001. *The Desktop Guide to Complementary and Alternative Medicine: an evidence based approach*. Mosby.

61 http://irweb.swmed.edu/newspub/newsdetl.asp?story_id = 312.

62 http://internet.citizens.coop/alexandertechnique/osteoporosis.htm

63 Ernst, E. (editor), 2001. *The Desktop Guide to Complementary and Alternative Medicine: an evidence based approach*. Mosby.

64 Raloff, Janet, 1999. Medicinal EMFs. *Science News*, 156, No. 20, November 13, 1999, 316.

65 http://www.osteo.org/osteo.html

66 Cummings, S. R., Nevitt, M. C., Browner, W. S. and others, 1995. Risk factors for hip fracture in white women: Study of Osteoporotic Fractures Research Group. *N E J of Med*, 332 (12), 767–773.

67 Cameron, Ian D. 2002. Hip protectors. *British Medical Journal*, 324, 16 February 2002 375–6.

68 http://www.icett.or.jp/lpca_jp.nsf/

69 see Plant, Jane, 2001. *Your Life in Your Hands*. Paperback edition. Virgin Books.

70 http://www.kanazawa-med.ac.jp/~ pubhealt/ikadai2/itaiitai-e/itai01.html

71 *Ibid.*

72 *Ibid.*

73 Dohi, Y. and six others, 1993. Effect of cadmium on osteogenesis within diffusion chambers by bone marrow cells: biochemical evidence of decreased bone formation capacity. *Toxicology and Applied Pharmacology*, 120, 2.

74 http://www.icsu-scope.org/cdmeeting/gochfeld%20abstract%20(1).htm

75 *Ibid.*

76 http://www.osha-slc.gov/SLTC/cadmium/

77 World Health Organisation, 1996. *Trace Elements in Human Nutrition and Health*. World Health Organisation.

78 Murray, J. J., Rugg-Gunn, A. J. and Jenkin, G. N., 1991. *Fluoride in Caries Prevention*. Third edition. Butterworth-Heinemann.

79 Zan-dao, W., Lin-ye, Z. and Ri-chuan, B., 1979. Endemic food borne fluorosis in Guizhou, China. *Chinese Journal of Preventive Medicine*, 13, 148–151.

80 Lee, John R., 1999. *Natural progesterone*. Second revised edition. Jon Carpenter.

81 World Health Organisation, 1996. *Trace Elements in Human Nutrition and Health*. World Health Organisation.

82 *Ibid.*

83 Lotz, M., Zisman, E. and Bartter, F. C., 1968. Evidence for a phosphorus-depletion syndrome in man. *N E J of Med*, 278, 409–415.

84 World Health Organisation, 1996. *Trace Elements in Human Nutrition and Health*. World Health Organisation.

85 *Ibid.*

86 Plant, J. 2001. *Your Life in Your Hands*. Paperback edition. Virgin Books.

87 Abraham, N. G., 1996. Hematopoietic effects of benzene inhalation assessed by long-term bone marrow culture. *Environmental Health Perspectives*, 104, Supplement 6, 1277–1282.

88 Plant, J. A. and Davis, D. L. 2003. Breast and Prostate cancer: sources and pathways of endocrine-disrupting chemicals (EDCs), in *Geology and Health*. Skinner, H. C. W. and Berger, A. R. (eds). Oxford University Press, 95–9.

89 The Royal Society, 2000. Endocrine-disrupting chemicals. *Document* 06/00. The Royal Society.

90 Sumpter, J. P. and Jobling, S., 1995. *Environmental Health Perspectives*, 103, 173–178.

91 Tylor, C. R. and Routledge, E. J., 1988. Natural and anthropogenic environmental oestrogens: the scientific basis for risk assessment. Oestrogenic effects in fish in English Rivers with evidence of their causation. *Pure and Applied Chemistry*, 70, 1795–1804.

92 *Ibid.*

93 Plant, Jane. 2001. *Your Life in Your Hands*. Paperback edition. Virgin Books.

94 The Royal Society, 2000. Endocrine-disrupting chemicals. *Document* 06/00. The Royal Society.

95 Retailers pledge to report on use of hazardous chemicals. *ENDS Report*, 331, August 2002, 31.

96 Reuters, 8 October 1998.

97 Pearson, J. K., 2000. *The Air Quality Challenge*. American Society of Automotive Engineers and HMSO.

Chapter 7: It's an Ill Wind that Blows No One Any Good

1 http://www.osteo.org/osteo.html (the website of the National Institutes of Health, Osteoporosis and Related Bone Diseases – National Resource Centre).

2 Ray, N. F., Chan, J. K., Thamer, M. and others, 1997. Medical expenditures for the treatment of osteoporotic fractures in the United States in 1995: report from the National Osteoporosis Foundation. *Journal of Bone and Mineral Research*, 12 (1), 24–35.

3 Melton, L. J. 3d, Thamer, M., Ray, N. F. and others, 1997. Fractures attributable to osteoporosis: report from the National Osteoporosis Foundation. *J Bone Miner Res*, 12 (1), 16–23.

4 Ray, N. F., Chan, J. K., Thamer, M. and others, 1997. Medical expenditures for the treatment of osteoporotic fractures in the United States in 1995: report from the National Osteoporosis Foundation. *J Bone Miner Res*, 12 (1), 24–35.

5 Melton, L. J. 3d, Thamer, M., Ray, N. F. and others, 1997. Fractures attributable to osteoporosis: report from the National Osteoporosis Foundation. *J Bone Miner Res*, 12 (1), 16–23.

6 Ray, N. F., Chan, J. K., Thamer, M. and others, 1997. Medical expenditures for the treatment of osteoporotic fractures in the United States in 1995: report from the National Osteoporosis Foundation. *J Bone Miner Res*, 12 (1), 24–35.

7 *Ibid*.

8 http://www.osteoporosis.ca/OSTEO/D01-01.html, the website of the Osteoporosis Society of Canada.

9 Priorities for prevention of osteoporosis. Bath. National Osteoporosis Society. 1994.

10 Dept of Health (UK) Advisory Group on Osteoporosis, Dept of Health 1994.

11 Advisory group for osteoporosis report. London. Dept of Health. 1995.

12 http://www.osteoporosis.ca/OSTEO/D01-01.html

13 http://www.osteofound.org/iof/index.html

14 http://www.osteofound.org/advocacy_policy/iof_statement.html

15 Robbins, John, 1987. *Diet for a New America*. Stillpoint Publishing.

16 Kradjian, R. D., 1994. *Save Yourself from Breast Cancer*. New York: Berkley Books.

17 http://www.afpafitness.com/milkdoc.htm

18 McDougall, John, 2000. *The McDougall Program for Women*.

19 http://www.milksucks.com/osteo.html

20 McDougall, John, 1985. *McDougall's Medicine*. New Century Publishing.

21 http://www.milksucks.com/osteo.html

22 Plant, Jane, 2000. *Your Life in Your Hands*. Paperback edition. Virgin Books.

23 Kradjian, R. D., 1994. *Save Yourself from Breast Cancer*. New York: Berkley Books.

24 Outwater, J. L., Nicholson, A. and Barnard, N., 1997. Dairy Products and Breast Cancer; the IGF, estrogen, and BGH hypothesis. *Medical Hypotheses*, 48, 453–461.

25 The European Commission. Health and Consumer Protection. Scientific Committee on Veterinary Measures Relating to Public Health – Outcome of Discussions, 1999. Report on Public Health Aspects of the Use of Bovine Somatotropin.

26 Pugh, R. H., 1981. Allergy to cow's milk protein. *Health Visitor*, 54, 231–233.

27 American Academy of Pediatrics Committee on Nutrition, 1992. The use of whole cow's milk in infancy. *Pediatrics*, 89, 1105–1109.

28 Anyon, C. P. and Clarkson, K. G., 1971. A cause of iron-deficiency anaemia in infants. *New Zealand Medical Journal*, 74, 24–25

29 Clyne, P. S. and Kulczycki, A., 1991. Human breast milk contains bovine IgG. Relationship to infant colic? *Pediatrics*, 87 (4), 439–444.

30 Wilson, J. F., Lahey, M. E. and Heiner, D. C., 1974. Studies on iron metabolism. V. Further observations on cow's-milk-induced gastrointestinal bleeding in infants with iron-deficiency anaemia. *Journal of Pediatrics*, 84, 335–344.

31 Pugh, R. H., 1981. Allergy to cow's milk protein. *Health Visitor*, 54, 231–233.

32 Bahna, S. L., 1987. Milk allergy in infancy. *Annals of Allergy*, 59, 131.

33 Scott, F. W., 1990. Cow milk and insulin-dependent diabetes mellitus: is there a relationship? *American Journal of Clinical Nutrition*, 51, 489–491.

34 The Institute of Food Science & Technology Position Statement, 1998. *Food Science & Technology Today*, 12 (4), 223–228, September. http://www.ifst.org/hottop23.html

35 *Financial Times* for the weekend 20–21 November 1999.

36 The Institute of Food Science & Technology Position Statement.

http://www.ifst.org/hottop2.html. Hard copies available from IFST, 5 Cambridge Court, 210 Shepherds Bush Road, London W6 7NJ.

37 Peter Martin, 2002. Milk: Nectar or Poison? *The Sunday Times Magazine*, July 21, 2002, 46–54.

38 Bristow, A. 2002. Organic processed food. *Which?* April 2002, 22–23.

39 *Ibid.*

40 Inside Story. *Which?* April 2002, 4.

41 Peter Martin, 2002. Milk: Nectar or Poison? *The Sunday Times Magazine*, July 21, 2002, 46–54.

42 www.thetareports.com

43 www.postgradmed.com/issues/1998/10_98/goddard.htm

44 *Ibid.*

45 Lee, John R., 1999. *Natural Progesterone*. Second revised edition. Jon Carpenter.

46 Proir, J. C. and Vigna, V. M., 1990. Spinal bone loss and ovulatory disturbances. *New England Journal of Medicine*, 323, 1221–1227.

47 Rudy, D. R., 1990. Hormone replacement therapy. *Postgraduate Medicine*, Dec 1990, 157–164.

48 http://www.milksucks.com/osteo.html

49 *The Practitioner*, Nov 95, Vol 239, 650.

50 Darwin, Charles, 1872. *The Origin of Species*. Sixth edition.

INDEX

A

acetic acid 42
acid-alkaline balance 34, 44, 61–6, 67–74, 99, 159–63
acidosis 43, 71
acids, properties of 42
additives, reducing 102
Advertising Standards Agency (ASA) 142, 143
aerosol spray 132
alcohol 20, 49, 58–9, 102, 112, 151
Alexander, Frederick 120
Alexander technique 120
alkalis, properties of 44
Alkalize or Die (Baroody) 71
alkalosis 39
alkyl pherols 129
allergies 109–12
aluminium 10, 127
animal protein 60–6, 149–50
anti-androgens 128
anti-inflammatory drugs (NSAIDs) 42
antioestrogens 17
apricots
    compote 165–6
    and pecan rum torte 276–7
artificial sweeteners 144
ascorbic acid 42
Asian noodle and watercress salad 192–3
asparagus
    couscous with peas and 211–12
    crab and asparagus soup 183
    leek, pea and asparagus risotto 214–15
aubergines
    aubergine and potato curry 255–6
    chickpeas with Moroccan 210–11
    spicy aubergine purée 204
avocado
    chilled avocado soup 180–1
    with ginger prawns 193–4
    with ginger vinaigrette 194–5
    and strawberry salad 193
    and tomato bruschetta 166
Ayurvedic medical system 155

B

Baby and Child Care (Spock) 141
bananas
    bread 167–8
    milk shake 166–7
Baroody, Theodore A. Jr 71
bean curd
    and mushroom soup 177
    with oyster sauces 209–10
    rolls 208–9

sesame, with snow peas and almonds 219–20
    and spinach soup 178
bean sprouts, stir-fried spinach and 265–6
beans, green beans with ginger 257–8
beetroot and orange salad 195
berry smoothie 168
bisphosphonates 16, 17, 148
black cohosh 115, 116
bok choy
    sautéed, with Worcester sauce 261–2
    stir-fried scallops with snow peas and 230–1
bones
    marrow 33
    matrix, calcification of 54, 55
    microfractures 33
    mineral density 14–16, 23, 52, 53, 55, 56
    mineralisation 17, 59
    remodelling 32–3
    skeleton 29, 30–1
boron 89, 90
bovine tuberculosis 141
breakfasts 165
breast cancer 22, 49, 113, 115
breast milk 55–6
brewer's yeast 107
British Geological Survey 65, 125
broccoli
    and lemon grass soup 178–9
    and potato soup 179–80
brucellosis 141
bruschetta, avocado and tomato 166
BSE 141
buffers 36, 43

C

cabbage, carrot and cabbage salad 205–6
cadmium 81, 87, 100, 123, 124–6, 129
cakes 276–8
calcitonin 17, 32, 148
calcium
    breast milk content 55–6
    in foods 56–7, 81, 82–3
    hip fracture incidence rates, link with 18, 23, 49–57, 75–7, 76, 106–7
    recommended intake 19, 53–7
    salts 17
    supplements 55, 106–7
    supply 18–23, 30–1, 106–7
    urinary loss 64
Campbell, Dr T. Colin 66, 147
Canadian Food Protection Branch 115
cancer *see* breast cancer; cervical cancer; endometrial cancer
carrot